2010 Protocols for Mosby's Virtual Patient Encounters

Use these protocols to replace those included in your VPE software. Updated to reflect the 2010 American Heart Association Guidelines for Cardiopulmonary Resuscitation and Emergency Cardiovascular Care.

Table of Contents

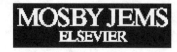

Acute Coronary Syndromes
(In the presence of chest pain with a suspected cardiac origin)

Emergency Medical Technician Level
- Follow General Supportive Care Protocol
- Follow General Airway Management Protocol if indicated
- Prepare to perform CPR and defibrillation if needed
- Evaluate oxygen saturation levels
    o If <94% administer oxygen 4 L/min*
- Assist ventilations if needed
- Administer aspirin
- Assist patient with nitroglycerin administration
- Request ALS assistance, if available
- Acquire and transmit 12-lead ECG, per local protocol

Advanced Emergency Medical Technician Level
- Establish IV access
- Administer nitroglycerin if indicated

Paramedic Level
- Monitor and interpret ECG
- Consider morphine sulfate if pain unrelieved by nitroglycerin
- Obtain and interpret 12-lead ECG
    o Interpret ST and T wave changes and injury patterns
    o Repeat as indicated to evaluate any changes
- If ST elevation myocardial infarction (STEMI) or new left bundle branch block (LBBB) identified
    o Consider triage to chest pain center per protocol
    o Determine eligibility for fibrinolytic treatment if indicated
        ▪ Prepare for fibrinolytic administration per local protocol

*American Heart Association. (2010). 2010 American Heart Association Guidelines for Cardiopulmonary Resuscitation and Emergency Cardiovascular Care. *Circulation, 122*(18 Supplement 3), S639-S946.

Altered Mental Status
(In the presence of suspected overdose or poisoning)

Emergency Medical Technician Level
- Follow General Supportive Care Protocol
- Follow General Airway Management Protocol
- Ventilate if needed
- Evaluate oxygen saturation level
- Administer supplemental oxygen
- Administer oral glucose as indicated for hypoglycemia if level of consciousness and ability to swallow permits
- Treat for shock
- Evaluate nature of substance ingested, inhaled, absorbed
- Consider trauma
- Consult with medical direction and poison control as indicated

Advanced Emergency Medical Technician Level
- Establish IV
  - Consider IO in child if critical and unable to establish IV
  - Administer fluid bolus if indicated for hypotension
- Evaluate blood glucose level
  - Administer dextrose 50% (or 25% or 10% based on age and protocol)
  - Administer glucagon if unable to establish vascular access
- Administer naloxone (Narcan) if suspected narcotic overdose
- If wheezing, consider bronchodilator

Paramedic Level
- Consider activated charcoal if ingestion less than 1 hour and adequate airway and adequate level of consciousness
- Consider IO if unable to establish IV
- If hypotension remains, repeat fluid bolus
- If seizures present, administer a benzodiazepine
- Consider and treat underlying cause if present:
  - Suspected TCA overdose
    - Consider sodium bicarbonate
  - Suspected β-blocker or calcium channel blocker overdose
    - Consider glucagon, atropine, calcium*
  - Suspected organophosphate/cabamate poisoning
    - Consider atropine
- Consider other causes of altered mental status
  - Digoxin toxicity
  - Drug abuse
  - Anaphylaxis
  - Carbon monoxide poisoning
  - Food poisoning
  - Stroke
  - Metabolic problems

*American Heart Association. (2010). 2010 American Heart Association Guidelines for Cardiopulmonary Resuscitation and Emergency Cardiovascular Care. *Circulation, 122*(18 Supplement 3), S639-S946.

Anaphylaxis
(In the presence of suspected allergic reaction)

Emergency Medical Technician Level
- Follow General Supportive Care Protocol
- Follow General Airway Management Protocol
- Evaluate oxygen saturation
- Administer high-concentration oxygen
- Assist ventilation if needed
- Assist with epinephrine autoinjector if available
- Treat for shock
- Reassess frequently
- Rapid transport and/or call for ALS intercept

Advanced Emergency Medical Technician Level
- Establish IV access and infuse IV fluids to treat shock
  - Establish IO in pediatric patient if unable to establish IV
- Administer epinephrine IM*
- Consider bronchodilator after epinephrine

Paramedic Level
- Establish IO if unable to establish IV
  - Continue fluid infusion for signs of shock
- Consider repeating epinephrine if indicated
- Consider antihistamine
- Consider corticosteroid
- Consider vasopressors

*American Heart Association. (2010). 2010 American Heart Association Guidelines for Cardiopulmonary Resuscitation and Emergency Cardiovascular Care. *Circulation, 122*(18 Supplement 3), S639-S946.

Acute Pulmonary Edema
(In the presence of difficulty breathing, and crackles [rales] and wheezing)

Emergency Medical Technician Level
- Follow General Supportive Care Protocol
- Follow General Airway Protocol
- Position patient
- Evaluate oxygen saturation levels
    o Administer high concentration oxygen
- Evaluate ventilation
    o Assist ventilation with bag-mask if indicated
- Acquire and transmit 12-lead ECG if available

Advanced Emergency Medical Technician Level
- Establish IV
- Administer nitroglycerin 0.4 mg tablet/spray if BP >90 mmHg
    o Repeat every 5 minutes to 3 doses maximum

Paramedic Level
- Apply continuous positive airway pressure
- Administer morphine 2-4 mg IV after nitroglycerin*
- Consider furosemide (if signs of fluid overload) if BP >90 mmHg*
- If signs of shock
    o Consider dobutamine (BP 70 to 100 mmHg)
    o Consider dopamine (BP <70 to 100 mmHg)
    o Consider norepinephrine (BP <70 mmHg)

*American Heart Association. (2010). 2010 American Heart Association Guidelines for Cardiopulmonary Resuscitation and Emergency Cardiovascular Care. *Circulation, 122*(18 Supplement 3), S639-S946.

Asystole/Pulseless Electrical Activity

Emergency Medical Technician Level
- Follow General Supportive Care Protocol
- Assess responsiveness
- Assess for absent or gasping breaths
- Call for help and AED
- Assess pulse for up to 10 seconds
- If no pulse, begin cycles of 30 chest compressions to 2 breaths
    - 15 chest compressions to 2 breaths when 2 rescuers present
- When AED arrives assess rhythm and if no shock advised
    - Resume CPR for 2 minutes then analyze rhythm
- Consider terminating resuscitation per protocol
- If return of spontaneous circulation (ROSC)
    - Maintain airway and ventilation
    - Assess vital signs
    - Administer oxygen to maintain SaO_2 $\geq$94%

Advanced Emergency Medical Technician Level
- Consider supraglottic airway
    - After initial CPR and rhythm analysis
- Insert IV

Paramedic Level
- Apply ECG monitor and defibrillator and assess ECG rhythm
- Continue CPR
- Insert IO if IV not established
- Administer epinephrine 1 mg IV/IO
    - Repeat every 3 to 5 minutes
    - May replace first or second dose of epinephrine with vasopressin 40 units IV/IO
- Consider endotracheal intubation
- Confirm placement per General Airway Policy
- Consider and treat reversible causes
- Consider terminating resuscitation per protocol
- If ROSC
    - Consider hypothermia protocol

Behavioral Emergencies
(In the presence of a change in mood or behavior that requires immediate attention)

Emergency Medical Technician Level
- Follow General Supportive Care Protocol
- Follow General Airway Management Protocol if indicated
- Evaluate SaO2 if indicated
- Apply oxygen if indicated
- Ventilate if indicated
- Seek possible causes for change in behavior
    o Medical cause
    o Psychiatric cause
- Physically restrain patient if indicated
- Notify law enforcement and poison control if indicated

Advanced Emergency Medical Technician Level
- Establish IV if indicated
- Measure blood glucose level if indicated
    o Administer dextrose if hypoglycemic
        ▪ Administer glucagon if IV cannot be established
- Consider narcotic antagonist if indicated

Paramedic Level
- Monitor ECG if indicated
- Consider the need for chemical restraints

Burns

Emergency Medical Technician Level
- Ensure personal safety
- Follow General Supportive Care Protocol
- Follow General Airway Protocol as needed
- Remove patient from the burning source
- Stop the burning process by removing clothing and jewelry or rinsing off chemicals
    - Consider cooling burns with copious amounts of room temperature water per local protocol*
    - Cover patient with dry, clean sheet after burning process stopped and maintain warmth with blankets
- Prepare to assist ventilations if indicated
- Estimate burn depth and size

Advanced Emergency Medical Technician Level
- Insert supraglottic airway if indicated
- Establish IV
    - Administer fluid using burn resuscitation formula such as the Parkland formula

Paramedic Level
- Monitor airway and perform endotracheal intubation if needed
- Consider inserting gastric tube (large burns)
- Consider monitoring ECG
- Consider pain managment

* Prehospital Trauma Life Support Committee of The National Association of Emergency Medical Technicians in Cooperation with The Committee on Trauma of the American College of Surgeons. (2011). *PHTLS Prehospital Trauma Life Support*. St. Louis: Mosby.

Environmental Emergencies, Hypothermia
(In the presence of signs/symptoms of abnormal thermoregulation)

Emergency Medical Technician Level
- Follow General Supportive Care Protocol
- Follow General Airway Management Protocol
- Remove all wet clothing; cover patient with warm blankets; turn on heat in patient compartment of ambulance
- Evaluate oxygen saturation (cold may impair assessment)
- Apply warm, humidified oxygen
- Assist ventilation if indicated
- Treat for shock
- Place heat packs (covered with towels) on neck, armpits, groin
- Handle gently
- Transport without delay

Advanced Emergency Medical Technician Level
- Assess core temperature if possible
- Establish IV
    o Infuse warmed IV fluids per protocol

Paramedic Level
- Monitor ECG
- Contact medical direction for pharmacologic orders

Environmental Emergencies, Hyperthermia
(In the presence of signs/symptoms of abnormal thermoregulation)

Emergency Medical Technician Level
- Follow General Supportive Care Protocol
- Move patient to a cool environment as soon as possible
- Follow General Airway Management Protocol
- Position responsive patient supine
    o Position unresponsive patient left lateral recumbent unless ventilation needed
- Evaluate oxygen saturation
- Administer oxygen
- Ventilate patient if indicated
- Measure temperature
- Remove clothing and cool patient with cool water spray*
- If alert with no vomiting, give patient cool electrolyte-carbohydrate drink

Advanced Emergency Medical Technician Level
- If unable to drink, establish IV
    o Administer IV fluids per protocol
    o Consider fluid challenge for hypotension

Paramedic Level
- Monitor ECG if serious signs and symptoms present
- Consider benzodiazepines to treat seizures
    - Or for severe shivering during cooling in unresponsive patients with advanced airway

Environmental Emergencies, Submersion/Drowning

Emergency Medical Technician Level
- Follow General Supportive Care Protocol
- Apply spinal immobilization if needed for trauma
- Follow General Airway Management Protocol
    - Prepare to suction
- Remove from water safely
- Evaluate oxygen saturation
- Ventilate if indicated
- Perform CPR if indicated
- Remove wet clothing and dry patient
    - Assess for hypothermia
    - Warm patient as in hypothermia protocol if indicated
- Rapid transport

Advanced Emergency Medical Technician Level
- Consider need for supraglottic airway
- Establish IV
- Consider nebulized beta-agonist if wheezing present

Paramedic Level
- Consider endotracheal intubation
- Monitor ECG
- Treat cardiac dysrhythmias according to AHA guidelines

* American Heart Association. (2010). 2010 American Heart Association Guidelines for Cardiopulmonary Resuscitation and Emergency Cardiovascular Care. *Circulation, 122*(18 Supplement 3), S639-S946.

General Airway Management
(In the presence of airway/ventilation compromise)

Emergency Medical Technician Level
- Perform manual maneuvers to open the airway if needed
- Consider
    - Suctioning the airway
    - Inserting an oropharyngeal device
    - Inserting a nasopharyngeal device

Advanced Emergency Medical Technician Level
- Insert a supraglottic airway if indicated*
- Confirm placement of supraglottic airway using multiple methods
    - Look for chest rise
    - Listen for presence of bilateral breath sounds
    - Listen for absence of bubbling in epigastrium during ventilation
    - End-tidal CO_2 detector
        - Capnography is most reliable†

Paramedic Level
- Consider drug-assisted intubation if indicated
- Insert an endotracheal tube if indicated
    - Orotracheal
    - Nasotracheal
- Confirm as above and may also consider
    - Direct visualization
    - Esophageal detector device
    - Other end-tidal CO_2 detector devices if capnography unavailable
        - Capnometry
        - Colorimetric
- If unable to intubate AND unable to ventilate
    - Translaryngeal cannula ventilation
    - Cricothyrotomy per protocol

---

* American Heart Association. (2010). 2010 American Heart Association Guidelines for Cardiopulmonary Resuscitation and Emergency Cardiovascular Care. *Circulation, 122*(18 Supplement 3), S639-S946.

† National EMS Scope of Practice

Hypertensive Disorders of Pregnancy

Emergency Medical Technician Level
- Follow General Supportive Care Protocol
- Follow General Airway Management Protocol
- Place patient in lateral recumbent position
- Monitor oxygen saturation
- Administer oxygen
- If seizure occurs, protect patient from physical harm
  - After seizure stops assure patient's airway
- Call for ALS intercept or rapid transport

Advanced Emergency Medical Technician Level
- Insert supraglottic airway if indicated
- Establish IV access as needed
- Consider dextrose 50% if hypoglycemic
  - Consider glucagon if unable to establish vascular access

Paramedic Level
- Perform endotracheal intubation if indicated
- Apply cardiac monitor
- If patient is eclamptic consider magnesium sulfate
- If seizures persist despite magnesium treatment, consult medical direction for advice to administer other anticonvulsants

Hypoglycemia
(In the presence of signs and symptoms of hypoglycemia)

Emergency Medical Technician Level
- Follow General Supportive Care Protocol
- Follow General Airway Management Protocol if indicated
- Evaluate oxygen saturation
- Administer oxygen if indicated
- Adminster oral glucose per protocol

Advanced Emergency Medical Technician Level
- Establish IV
  - o Consider IO in pediatric patient if unable to establish IV based on patient condition and response to glucagon
- Evaluate blood glucose level
  - o Administer dextrose (50%, 25% or 10% per protocol)
  - o Administer glucagon if unable to establish IV

Paramedic Level
- Consider IO if unable to establish IV and patient does not respond to glucagon administration

Irregular Tachycardia

Emergency Medical Technician Level
- Follow General Supportive Care Protocol
- Follow Airway Management Protocol if indicated
- Assess responsiveness
- Perform primary assessment
    - Support airway and ventilation if patient cannot maintain
    - Administer oxygen if indicated
- Call for ALS intercept or rapid transport

Advanced Emergency Medical Technician Level
- Perform secondary assessment
- Establish IV access

Paramedic Level
- Apply ECG monitor and interpret ECG rhythm
    - Note whether the QRS complex is wide or narrow
    - Confirm that the tachycardia is irregular
- Determine whether the patient has serious signs or symptoms related to the tachycardia (stable or unstable?)
- Obtain and review 12-lead ECG to confirm origin of rhythm
- If unstable, irregular and narrow QRS complex–
    - Synchronized cardioversion*
        - 120 to 200 J biphasic; 200 J monophasic*
        - Repeat at same or higher dose if needed
- If unstable, irregular and wide QRS complex
    - Unsynchronized cardioversion at defibrillation dose
        - 120 to 200 J biphasic (per mfr); 360 J monophasic*
        - Repeat at same or higher dose if needed
- If stable and irregular narrow QRS complex
    - Consider βblocker or calcium channel blocker (consult medical direction)
- If stable and irregular wide complex
    - Consider procainamide or amiodarone infusion

- Differential Diagnosis
    - Search for and treat irreversible causes

* American Heart Association. (2010). 2010 American Heart Association Guidelines for Cardiopulmonary Resuscitation and Emergency Cardiovascular Care. *Circulation, 122*(18 Supplement 3), S639-S946.

Narrow-QRS Tachycardia with Regular Rhythm
(Regular ventricular rhythm)

Emergency Medical Technician Level
- Follow General Supportive Care Protocol
- Assess responsiveness
- Perform primary assessment
  - Support airway and ventilation if patient cannot maintain
  - Administer oxygen if indicated
- Call for ALS intercept or rapid transport

Advanced Emergency Medical Technician Level
- Perform advanced airway maneuvers if indicated
- Establish IV

Paramedic Level
- Monitor and interpret ECG
- Obtain 12-lead ECG if further information needed
- Stable narrow-QRS tachycardia
  - Sinus tachycardia
    - Find and treat underlying cause
  - SVT
    - Vagal maneuvers*
    - Adenosine 6 mg rapid IV (follow with NS flush)*
      - Repeat adenosine at 12 mg in 1 to 2 minutes if indicated*
    - β blocker or calcium channel blocker*
- Unstable narrow-QRS tachycardia
  - Sinus tachycardia – find and treat underlying cause
  - SVT
    - Consider sedation
    - Synchronized cardioversion*

---

* American Heart Association. (2010). 2010 American Heart Association Guidelines for Cardiopulmonary Resuscitation and Emergency Cardiovascular Care. *Circulation, 122*(18 Supplement 3), S639-S946.

Pediatric Cardiac Arrest

Emergency Medical Technician Level
- Assess responsiveness
- Assess for absent or gasping breaths
- Call for help and AED
- Assess pulse for up to 10 seconds
- If no pulse, begin cycles of 30 chest compressions to 2 breaths
    - 15 chest compressions to 2 breaths when 2 rescuers present
- When AED arrives assess rhythm and defibrillate if indicated
    - Use pediatric attenuator pads if available
    - Use defibrillator if available for infants <1 year
        - If defibrillator unavailable, use AED
    - Defibrillate if indicated
- Resume CPR immediately after defibrillation
- Reassess pulse and analyze rhythm every 2 minutes
    - Defibrillate if indicated
- If return of spontaneous circulation (ROSC)
    - Maintain airway and ventilation
    - Assess vital signs
    - Administer oxygen to maintain $SaO_2 \geq 94\%$

Advanced Emergency Medical Technician Level
- During arrest
    - Establish IV/IO access
    - Consider advanced airway
    - Consider reversible causes of arrest

Paramedic Level
- Apply ECG monitor and analyze ECG rhythm
- During arrest
    - After initial 2 minutes of CPR
        - Defibrillation if indicated at 2 J/kg (first shock)*
        - Administer epinephrine IV/IO 0.01 mg/kg*
    - Continue CPR for 2 minutes
    - Assess ECG rhythm
        - If ventricular fibrillation/ventricular tachycardia defibrillate 4 J/kg (second and subsequent shocks)
        - Resume CPR after shock
        - Administer amiodarone IV/IO 5 mg/kg*
- If ROSC consider hypothermia per local protocol

*American Heart Association. (2010). 2010 American Heart Association Guidelines for Cardiopulmonary Resuscitation and Emergency Cardiovascular Care. *Circulation, 122*(18 Supplement 3), S639-S946.

Respiratory Distress
(In the presence of wheezing with a history of asthma/COPD)

Emergency Medical Technician Level
- Follow General Supportive Care Protocol
- Assess and maintain airway
- Place patient in position of comfort
- Apply pulse oximeter
- Administer high-concentration oxygen
- Request ALS intercept if available
- Consider patient-assisted metered-dose inhaler

Advanced Emergency Medical Technician Level
- Insert a supraglottic airway if indicated
- Administer inhaled β agonist (repeat per local protocol)

Paramedic Level
- Consider continuous positive airway pressure if indicated
- Consider endotracheal intubation
- Consider corticosteroids
- Consider epinephrine*
- Consider magnesium

* American Heart Association. (2010). 2010 American Heart Association Guidelines for Cardiopulmonary Resuscitation and Emergency Cardiovascular Care. *Circulation, 122*(18 Supplement 3), S639-S946.

Symptomatic Bradycardia

Emergency Medical Technician Level
- Follow General Supportive Care Protocol
- Follow Airway Management Protocol if indicated
- Assist ventilation if indicated
- Assess oxygen saturation
- Administer oxygen if indicated

Advanced Emergency Medical Technician Level
- Establish IV if patient unstable

Paramedic Level
- Monitor ECG and determine rhythm
- Perform 12-lead ECG if it doesn't delay treatment
- If stable
    o Monitor and reassess
- If unstable*
    o Administer atropine 0.5 mg IV (repeat every 3 to 5 minutes)*
        ▪ Not effective in type II second-degree AV block or third-degree AV block with wide QRS
    o Attempt transcutaneous pacing
    o If no improvement after initial measures
        ▪ Consider dopamine infusion at 2 to 10 mcg/kg/min
                Or
        • Consider epinephrine infusion at 2 to 10 mcg/min

* American Heart Association. (2010). 2010 American Heart Association Guidelines for Cardiopulmonary Resuscitation and Emergency Cardiovascular Care. *Circulation, 122*(18 Supplement 3), S639-S946.

Seizure
(In the presence of altered consciousness or signs/symptoms of abnormal brain function)

Emergency Medical Technician Level
- Follow General Supportive Care Protocol
- Follow General Airway Management Protocol
    o Do not attempt to place anything in patient's mouth during tonic-clonic seizure
        - Administer oxygen
        - Evaluate oxygen saturation level
        - After seizure
            o Place in lateral recumbent position

Advanced Emergency Medical Technician Level
- Establish IV access
    o Consider IO in pediatric patient based on level of consciousness and response to glucagon
- Evaluate blood glucose level
    o Administer dextrose (50%, 25%, 10% per protocol) if hypoglycemic
        - Administer glucagon if unable to obtain IV

Paramedic Level
- Monitor and interpret ECG
- If active seizures administer anticonvulsant*
- Consider administration of naloxone
- For pregnant eclamptic patient administer magnesium sulfate per protocol*

* Sanders, M. (2011) Mosby's Paramedic Textbook, Elsevier, St. Louis.

Sexual Assault
(In the presence of any suspected sexual assault)

Emergency Medical Technician Level
- Call police if scene unsafe
    - Police contact in other situations may require patient consent depending on state law and local protocol
- Follow General Supportive Care Protocol
- Follow General Airway Protocol if indicated
- Evaluate oxygen saturation if indicated
- Administer oxygen if indicated
- Treat any noted trauma per trauma protocol
    - Examine genitalia only if significant bleeding is present
- Document patient statements and injuries in detail
- When possible have same gender caregiver perform history and exam
- Remain nonjudgmental
    - Avoid direct questions related to details of the sexual assault
- Preserve evidence from the crime scene (even if patient states they do not wish to press charges)
    - Disturb minor injuries as little as possible
    - Handle clothing minimally
    - Do not clean wounds unless absolutely necessary
    - Do not allow the patient to bathe, urinate, douche, drink, or brush teeth if possible
    - Bag blood-stained or soiled clothing in paper (not plastic) bags
    - Maintain chain of evidence

Advanced Emergency Medical Technician Level
- Establish IV if indicated
    - Administer IV fluids if signs of shock
- Consider pain management

Stroke
(In the presence of suspected interruption of blood flow to the brain)

Emergency Medical Technician Level
- Follow General Supportive Care Protocol
- Follow General Airway Management Protocol if indicated
- Perform immediate assessment
    - Assess Cincinnati Stroke Scale
    - Establish time of onset of stroke signs (last time known well)
- Evaluate oxygen saturation
    - Administer oxygen if SaO_2 <94%*
- Protect paralyzed extremities
- Provide comfort and support
- Transport to closest appropriate facility without delay
    - Notify hospital of possible stroke enroute

Advanced Emergency Medical Technician Level
- Establish IV access
- Evaluate blood glucose level and if hypoglycemic
    - Administer dextrose (50%, 25%, 10% per local protocol)
    - Administer glucagon if unable to establish IV

---

* American Heart Association. (2010). 2010 American Heart Association Guidelines for Cardiopulmonary Resuscitation and Emergency Cardiovascular Care. *Circulation, 122*(18 Supplement 3), S639-S946.

Trauma
(In the presence of any injury resulting from blunt or penetrating forces)

Emergency Medical Technician Level
- For suspected spinal trauma, apply manual spinal immobilization
- Follow General Supportive Care Protocol
- Follow General Airway Management Protocol if indicated
- Evaluate oxygen saturation
    o Administer oxygen if indicated
- Assist ventilation if indicated
- Treat for shock if present
- For flail segment with respiratory compromise
    o Assist ventilation with bag-mask and 100% oxygen
- For open pneumothorax
    o Apply occlusive dressing
- For traumatic brain injury
    o Assess GCS
- For penetrating trauma
    o Stabilize foreign objects
        ▪ Remove if in cheek and causing bleeding
- For fractures, sprains, and strains
    o Immobilize affected area including joint and/or bone above and below injury
        ▪ Apply ice, elevate extremity
- Transport to closest appropriate facility

Advanced Emergency Medical Technician Level
- Establish IV access
    o Infuse fluid to maintain systolic BP of 80 to 90 mmHg*
    o Consider pain management (per protocol if indicated)
    o Consider IO access in unresponsive critical pediatric patient if unable to establish IV

Paramedic Level
- Establish IO if patient is critical and unable to establish IV
- For tension pneumothorax
    o Perform needle chest decompression
- For hemothorax or pericardial tamponade
    o Treat for shock
- Administer IV analgesics as indicated

---

* Prehospital Trauma Life Support Committee of The National Association of Emergency Medical Technicians in Cooperation with The Committee on Trauma of the American College of Surgeons. (2011). *PHTLS Prehospital Trauma Life Support*. St. Louis: Mosby.

Pulseless Ventricular Tachycardia (VT)/Ventricular Fibrillation (VF)

Emergency Medical Technician Level
- Follow General Supportive Care Protocol
- Assess responsiveness
- Assess for absent or gasping breaths
- Call for help and AED
- Assess pulse for up to 10 seconds
- If no pulse, begin cycles of 30 chest compressions to 2 breaths*
    - When AED arrives assess rhythm and defibrillate if indicated
    - Resume CPR for 2 minutes
    - Assess rhythm and shock every 2 minutes if indicated
- If return of spontaneous circulation (ROSC)
    - Maintain airway and ventilation
    - Assess vital signs
    - Administer oxygen to maintain SaO_2 greater than or equal to 94%

Advanced Emergency Medical Technician Level
- Ensure quality CPR
- Establish IV
- Consider supraglottic airway after initial CPR and defibrillation (if indicated)
- Consider reversible causes

Paramedic Level
- Ensure quality CPR
    - Establish IO if needed
- Apply monitor/defibrillator and interpret VF/VT
    - Defibrillate at 120 to 200 J biphasic (based on manufacturer; repeat at); 360 J monophasic
    - Resume CPR for 2 minutes
        - Administer epinephrine 1 mg IV/IO *
            - Repeat every 3 to 5 minutes
            - May replace first or second dose of epinephrine with vasopressin 40 units IV/IO
    - Consider endotracheal intubation
        - Confirm per General Airway Management Protocol
            - Monitor capnography continuously if available
    - Reassess rhythm and pulse
    - Defibrillate
    - Resume CPR for 2 minutes
        - Administer amiodarone 5 mg/kg IV/IO*
        - Treat reversible causes
- If ROSC
    - Consider therapeutic hypothermia (per local protocol)*

---

* American Heart Association. (2010). 2010 American Heart Association Guidelines for Cardiopulmonary Resuscitation and Emergency Cardiovascular Care. *Circulation, 122*(18 Supplement 3), S639-S946.

Wide-QRS Tachycardia
(Regular Ventricular Rhythm with a pulse)

Emergency Medical Technician Level
- Follow General Supportive Care Protocol
- Follow General Airway Management Protocol
- Assess responsiveness
- Assess for breathing
  - Assist ventilation if indicated
- Assess pulse
- Determine blood pressure
- Measure oxygen saturation
  - Administer oxygen if indicated
- Request ALS intercept if available

Advanced Emergency Medical Technician Level
- Establish IV

Paramedic Level
- Monitor ECG and determine rhythm
- Perform 12-lead ECG if it doesn't delay treatment
- If stable
  - Consider adenosine if regular and monomorphic
  - Consider antiarrhythmic infusion
    - Procainamide 20 to 50 mg/min (until rhythm suppressed, QRS increases more than 50%, hypotension or maximum dose 17 mg/kg)
    - Amiodarone 150 mg IV over 10 minutes
      - Maintenance infusion 1 mg/min for first 6 hours
- If unstable
  - Consider sedation
  - Perform synchronized cardioversion 100 J
    - If rhythm is unchanged repeat per manufacturers recommendations

* American Heart Association. (2010). 2010 American Heart Association Guidelines for Cardiopulmonary Resuscitation and Emergency Cardiovascular Care. *Circulation, 122*(18 Supplement 3), S639-S946.

Virtual Patient Encounters

for

Henry/Stapleton: EMT Prehospital Care

Fourth Edition, Revised Reprint

Virtual Patient Encounters

for

Henry/Stapleton:
EMT Prehospital Care
Fourth Edition, Revised Reprint

Study guide prepared by
Kim D. McKenna, RN, BSN, CEN, EMT-P
Director of Education
St. Charles County Ambulance District
St. Peters, Missouri

Software developed by
Wolfsong Informatics, LLC
Tucson, Arizona

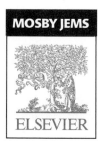

MOSBY JEMS

ELSEVIER

MOSBY JEMS
ELSEVIER

11830 Westline Industrial Drive
St. Louis, Missouri 63146

VIRTUAL PATIENT ENCOUNTERS
FOR HENRY/STAPLETON: EMT PREHOSPITAL CARE,
FOURTH EDITION

ISBN: 978-0-323-08675-2

Notice

Knowledge and best practice in this field are constantly changing. As new research and experience broaden our knowledge, changes in practice, treatment and drug therapy may become necessary or appropriate. Readers are advised to check the most current information provided (i) on procedures featured or (ii) by the manufacturer of each product to be administered, to verify the recommended dose or formula, the method and duration of administration, and contraindications. It is the responsibility of the practitioner, relying on their own experience and knowledge of the patient, to make diagnoses, to determine dosages and the best treatment for each individual patient, and to take all appropriate safety precautions. To the fullest extent of the law, neither the Publisher nor the Author assumes any liability for any injury and/or damage to persons or property arising out of or related to any use of the material contained in this book.

ISBN: 978-0-323-08675-2

Publishing Director: Andrew Allen
Managing Editor: Laura Bayless
Publishing Services Manager: Patricia Tannian
Project Manager: Sarah Wunderly
Cover Designer: Mark Oberkrom

Printed in United States of America

Last digit is the print number: 9 8 7 6 5 4 3 2 1

Contents

*Summative lesson—see "Orientation to *Virtual Patient Encounters*" for explanation.

Summative Lessons Listed by Case

Case 1: 20-year-old male—difficulty breathing (Lesson 14)

Case 2: 56-year-old female—fell (Lesson 12)

Case 3: 7-year-old female—seizure (Lesson 25)

Case 4: 64-year-old male – unknown medical (Lesson 13)

Case 5: 40-year-old male—vomiting blood (Lesson 21)

Case 6: 16-year-old female—unknown medical (Lesson 15)

Case 7: 8-year-old male—submersion (Lesson 16)

Case 8: 38-year-old male—suicide attempt (Lesson 18)

Case 9: 22-year-old female—assault (Lesson 23)

Case 10: 25-year-old female—abdominal pain (Lesson 20)

Case 11: 32-year-old male—gunshot wounds (Lesson 22)

Case 12: 57-year-old male—man down (Lesson 17)

Case 13: 5-month-old male—unresponsive (Lesson 24)

Case 14: 65-year-old male—difficulty breathing (Lesson 27)

Case 15: 42-year-old male—difficulty breathing (Lesson 11)

Acknowledgments

Virtual Patient Encounters was developed over 3 years with input from many emergency medical services (EMS) instructors around the United States, who participated in some fashion or another. Some traveled across the country to share their vision of what a valuable critical-thinking product would be; others wrote cases and recommended management sequences; some provided their expertise at focus groups and user-centered design studies; and many, many instructors reviewed the software, study guide, and implementation manual.

We are deeply grateful to each of you for helping us make this study guide a reality. Your education, dedication, and experience clearly shine through in this one-of-a-kind educational product for EMT students everywhere. Recognizing your contributions wherever you were involved—in the software, the study guide, and the implementation manual—does not truly express our gratitude.

I would like to offer a very special thank you to three of the best instructors in EMS who worked tirelessly creating this product and graciously made the many changes recommended by other subject matter experts: Twink Dalton, whose creative juices were never-ending, and John Gosford, whose field experience and technical expertise brought road-ready reality into each case. You two were a dynamic duo. Your shining lights were bright even on the dreariest of days, and your energy and enthusiasm were contagious. A special thank you is also extended to Kim McKenna, who thought it would be so much fun to write the study guide and implementation manual. Your determination to see this project through to its completion, even when the task was arduous and seemed overwhelming, delivered a finished product that is nothing short of genius. We are deeply indebted to each of you and owe you a large replacement supply of midnight oil.

To EMT instructors: I hope *Virtual Patient Encounters* fills in the frustrating gap of trying to prepare students to be critical thinkers and make the right clinical decisions for their patients before they enter their clinical experiences and the field.

To every EMT student who uses *Virtual Patient Encounters*: I hope this product brings you a valuable educational experience that prepares you for the real world of EMS. I wish you much success and compassion.

Linda Honeycutt
Executive Editor

Study Guide Contributors

David K. Anderson, BS, EMT-P
Program Director
NW Regional Training Center
Vancouver, Washington

Peter Connick, EMT-P, EMT I/C
Captain
Chatham Fire Rescue
Chatham, Massachusetts

Adjunct Faculty
Cape Cod Community College
West Barnstable, Massachusetts

Jon Cooper, NREMT-P
Lieutenant
Baltimore City Fire and EMS Academy
Baltimore, Maryland

John Gosford, BS, EMT-P
Associate Professor and EMS Coordinator
Lake City Community College
Lake City, Florida

Study Guide Reviewers

Kim Bemenderfer, NREMT-I, BS
EMS Educator
North Memorial EMS Education
Robbinsdale, Minnesota

Jon Cooper, NREMT-P
Lieutenant
Baltimore City Fire and EMS Academy
Baltimore, Maryland

Orlando J. Dominguez, Jr., MBA, FF/Paramedic
Chief of EMS/PIO
Brevard County Fire Rescue
Rockledge, Florida

Ann Maureen Dunphy, BS, EMT-I, WEMT
EMS Instructor
Eagle River Memorial Hospital
Eagle River, Wisconsin

Nicolet Area Technical College
Rhinelander, Wisconsin

Wilderness Medical Associates
Portland, Maine

Janet Fitts, RN, BSN, CEN, TNS, EMT-P
Educational Consultant
Prehospital Emergency Medical Education
Pacific, Missouri

Marguerite X. Haaga
Paramedic, Education Manager
The Center for Public Safety Education
East Berlin, Connecticut

Mark Milliron, MPA, MS, EMT-Instructor
Instructor in Health Policy and Administration
The Pennsylvania State University
University Park, Pennsylvania

Jason J. Zigmont, BS, NREMT-P, EMS-I
Executive Director
The Center for Public Safety Education
East Berlin, Connecticut

Getting Started

Getting Set Up

SYSTEM REQUIREMENTS

WINDOWS®

- Windows® PC
- Windows XP and Windows Vista
- Pentium® processor (or equivalent) @ 1 GHz (2 GHz or greater is recommended)
- 1.5 GB hard disk space
- 512 MB of RAM (1 GB or more is recommended)
- CD-ROM drive
- 800 × 600 screen size
- Thousands of colors
- Soundblaster 16 soundcard compatibility
- Stereo speakers or headphones

MACINTOSH®

Virtual Patient Encounters is not compatible with the Macintosh platform.

INSTALLATION INSTRUCTIONS

WINDOWS®

1. Insert the *Virtual Patient Encounters* CD-ROM.
2. Inserting the CD should automatically bring up the set-up screen if the current product is not already installed.
   a. If the set-up screen does not automatically appear (and *Virtual Patient Encounters* has not been already installed), navigate to the **My Computer** icon on your desktop or in your **Start** menu.

    b. Double-click on your CD-ROM drive.

    c. If installation does not start at this point:

       (1) Click the **Start** icon on the task bar, and select the **Run** option.

       (2) Type d:\setup.exe (where "d:\" is your CD-ROM drive), and press **OK**.

       (3) Follow the onscreen instructions for installation.

  3. Follow the onscreen instructions during the set-up process.

HOW TO LAUNCH *VIRTUAL PATIENT ENCOUNTERS*

WINDOWS®

1. Double-click on the **Virtual Patient Encounters BLS** icon located on your desktop.

2. *(alternative)* Navigate to the program via the Windows **Start** menu.

SCREEN SETTINGS

For best results, your computer monitor resolution should be set at a minimum of 800 × 600. The number of colors displayed should be set to "thousands or higher" (High Color or 16-bit) or "millions of colors" (True Color or 24-bit).

WINDOWS®

1. From the Start menu, select **Settings**, then **Control Panel**.

2. Double-click on the **Display** icon.

3. Click on the **Settings** tab.

4. Under **Screen Resolution**, use the slider bar to select **800 × 600 pixels**.

5. Access the **Colors** drop-down menu by clicking on the down arrow.

6. Select **High Color (16-bit)** or **True Color (24-bit)**.

7. Click on **OK**.

8. You may be asked to verify the setting changes. Click **Yes**.

9. You may be asked to restart your computer to accept the changes. Click **Yes**.

TECHNICAL SUPPORT

Technical support for this product is available between 7:30 AM and 7:00 PM (CST), Monday through Friday. Before calling, be sure your computer meets the recommended system requirements to run this software. Inside the United States, call 1-800-692-9010. Outside the United States, call 1-314-447-8094. You may also fax your questions to 1-314-447-8078 or via e-mail at: technical.support@elsevier.com.

■ Accessing the *Virtual Patient Encounters Online Study Guide* on Evolve

The product you have purchased is part of the Evolve family of online courses and learning resources. Read the following information thoroughly to get started. To access the *Virtual Patient Encounters Online Study Guide* on Evolve, your instructor will provide you with the username and password needed to access the *Virtual Patient Encounters Online Study Guide* on the Evolve Learning System. Once you have received this information, follow these instructions:

1. Go to the Evolve login page (http://evolve.elsevier.com/login).

Trademarks: Windows, Pentium, and America Online are registered trademarks.

2. Enter your username and password in the **Login to My Evolve** area and click the arrow or hit **Enter**.

3. You will be taken to your personalized **My Evolve** page, where the course will be listed under the banner titled **Courses**.

TECHNICAL REQUIREMENTS

To use the *Virtual Patient Encounters Online Study Guide*, you will need access to a computer that is connected to the Internet and equipped with web browser software that supports frames. For optimal performance, speakers and a high-speed Internet connection are recommended. However, slower dial-up modems (56 K minimum) are acceptable.

WEB BROWSERS

Supported web browsers include Microsoft Internet Explorer (IE), version 6.0 or higher, and Mozilla Firefox, version 1.5 or higher.

If you use America Online (AOL) for web access, you will need AOL, version 4.0 or higher, and IE, version 5.0 or higher. Do not use earlier versions of AOL with earlier versions of IE because you will have difficulty accessing many features.

For best results with AOL:

- Connect to the Internet using AOL, version 4.0 or higher.
- Open a private chat in AOL (this allows the AOL client to remain open without asking whether you wish to disconnect while minimized).
- Minimize AOL.
- Launch a recommended browser.

Whichever browser you use, the browser preferences must be set to enable cookies and JavaScript, and the cache must be set to reload every time.

ENABLE COOKIES

Browser	Steps
Internet Explorer (IE), version 6.0 or higher	1. Select **Tools → Internet Options**. 2. Select **Privacy** tab. 3. Use the slider (slide down) to **Accept All Cookies**. 4. Click **OK**. *OR* 3. Click the **Advanced** button. 4. Click the checkbox next to **Override Automatic Cookie Handling**. 5. Click the **Accept** radio buttons under **First-Party Cookies and Third-Party Cookies**. 6. Click **OK**.
Mozilla Firefox, version 1.5 or higher	1. Select **Tools → Internet Options**. 2. Select the **Privacy** icon. 3. Click to expand **Cookies**. 4. Select **Allow** sites to set cookies. 5. Click **OK**.

SET CACHE TO ALWAYS RELOAD A PAGE

Browser	Steps
Internet Explorer (IE), version 6.0 or higher	1. Select **Tools** → **Internet Options**. 2. Select **General** tab. 3. Go to the **Temporary Internet Files**, and click the **Settings** button. 4. Select the radio button for **Every visit to the page**, and click **OK** when complete.
Mozilla Firefox, version 2.0 or higher	1. **Select Tools** → **Options**. 2. Select the **Privacy** icon. 3. Click to expand **Cache**. 4. Set the value to "**0**" in the **Use up to: ___ MB of disk space for the cache** field. 5. Click **OK**.

PLUG-INS

 Adobe Acrobat Reader—With the free Acrobat Reader software, you can view and print Adobe PDFs. Many Evolve products offer student and instructor manuals, checklists, and more in the PDF format!
Download at: http://www.adobe.com

 Apple QuickTime—Install this software to hear word pronunciations, heart and lung sounds, and many other helpful audio clips in the Evolve Online Courses!
Download at: http://www.apple.com

 Adobe Flash Player—This player will enhance your viewing of many Evolve web pages, as well as educational short- to long-form animation in the Evolve Learning System!
Download at: http://www.adobe.com

 Adobe Shockwave Player—Shockwave is best for viewing the many interactive learning activities in Evolve Online Courses!
Download at: http://www.adobe.com

 Microsoft Word Viewer—With this viewer, Microsoft Word users can share documents with those who do not have Word, and users without Word can open and view Word documents. Many Evolve products have test banks, student and instructor manuals, and other documents available for downloading and viewing on your own computer!
Download at: http://www.microsoft.com

 Microsoft PowerPoint Viewer—View PowerPoint 97, 2000, and 2002 presentations with this viewer, even if you do not have PowerPoint. Many Evolve products have slides available for downloading and viewing on your own computer!
Download at: http://www.microsoft.com

SUPPORT INFORMATION

Live support is available to customers in the United States and Canada from 7:30 AM to 7:00 PM (CST), Monday through Friday, by calling **1-800-401-9962**. You can also send an e-mail to evolve-support@elsevier.com.

In addition, **24/7 support information** is available on the Evolve web site (http://evolve.elsevier.com) including:

- Guided tours
- Tutorials
- Frequently asked questions (FAQs)
- Online copies of course user guides
- And much more!

Orientation to *Virtual Patient Encounters*

Welcome to *Virtual Patient Encounters!*

The course of study to become an emergency medical technician (EMT) is complex and involves not only a narrow look at a specific topic, but being an EMT also requires that you have a broad foundation of knowledge to enable you to provide effective and safe patient care. Sometimes discrimination among similar choices is required. In the textbooks, patient presentation offers only a clear, one-faceted look at each illness or injury. When reading, patient care may seem similarly straightforward and the path to the correct decisions and interventions may appear very clear. In contrast, real patient situations are often fuzzy, complex, and confusing. This combination of study guide with simulation software is designed to help you bridge the gap between the books and the street and to assist you in "putting it all together." We hope you will reflect on the knowledge from each of the foundation chapters when you evaluate and treat these patients. It is our goal that this course of study will make your transition to the field easier and will give you the confidence to make the right decisions when they matter the most.

BEFORE YOU START

For best results, use the *Virtual Patient Encounters* simulation software as directed by the lessons found in this study guide. Each lesson begins with a reading assignment, usually a single chapter in your textbook. Make sure to read this material before beginning the lesson because you will need to understand the concepts before attempting to answer the questions in the study guide or before you make any patient care decisions in the software. Some lessons also list "relevant" chapters in addition to the reading assignment. These *summative* lessons will require a broad understanding of many concepts from different topic areas before being attempted. We highly recommend that you read all these relevant chapters in addition to the reading assignment before attempting the summative lessons.

The following icons are used throughout the study guide to help you quickly identify particular activities and assignments:

Reading Assignment—Tells you which textbook chapter(s) you should read before starting each lesson.

Writing Activity—Certain activities focus on written responses such as filling out forms or completing documentation.

 CD-ROM Activity—Marks the beginning of an activity that uses the *Virtual Patient Encounters* simulation software.

 Reference—Indicates questions and activities that require you to consult your textbook.

 Time—Indicates the approximate amount of time needed to complete the exercise.

Each lesson in the study guide provides specific directions that explain what to do in the software to prepare for each exercise. These directions are always bulleted and are always indicated by an arrow (→) in the left margin. Do no more or no less than what the directions indicate. For example, many lessons require that you watch only a video before answering the study guide questions, whereas others will direct you to also perform your primary assessment in the software. Summative lessons will direct you to care for the patient from beginning to end as best you can, based on what you have learned from the textbook and in class.

Although the study guide lessons provide specific directions as to what to do in the software, when it comes to caring for the patients (e.g., performing assessments and interventions), you will need to understand what all the buttons do. The following orientation will explain the entire software interface and how you can treat each of the 15 cases.

HOW TO LOG IN

To open the *Virtual Patient Encounters* simulation program, you can either double click the *Virtual Patient Encounters BLS* icon that should appear on your computer desktop after you have installed the software, or you can click on **Start**, then **Programs**, then **Virtual Patient Encounters**, then **Virtual Patient Encounters BLS**. Once the program begins, you will see an anti-piracy warning and a video montage before the log-on screen appears (shown below). If you wish to skip the video montage, click on the **Skip Intro** button at the bottom of the screen.

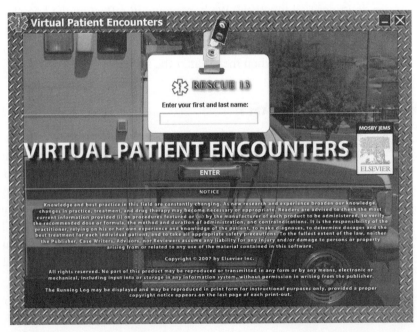

Type your first and last name into the name tag pictured, and click **Enter**. This will take you to a list of all 15 cases in this program (shown in the first screen on the following page).

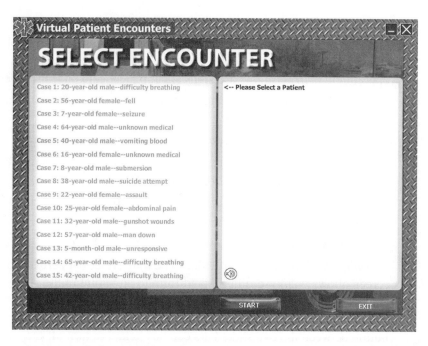

Once you click on a patient, you can listen to the dispatch report, which will also appear as text in the panel on the right side of the screen. (If you don't want to hear the dispatch audio, you can click on the **MUTE** icon.) After you have listened to and read the dispatch information, you can then click **START** to respond to the case. (An **EXIT** button also appears on this screen if you want to close the entire program.)

Once you select a case, your initial approach to the scene and patient will play in a video. All the videos include an overview of the area from the perspective of the ambulance (shown below) to enable you to think about staging considerations and scene safety.

On approaching the patient, you will have an opportunity to perform the scene size-up, form an initial visual impression of the patient, and listen to information provided by conscious patients and any first responders, family members, or bystanders on the scene. Be aware that

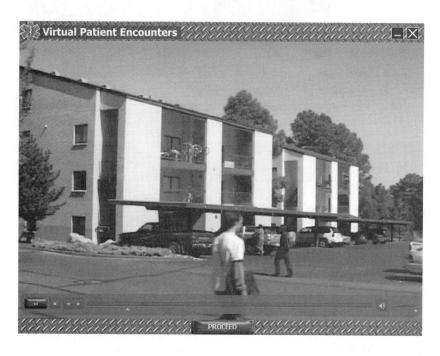

some videos intentionally deviate from "best practice" to give you a chance to critique how things were handled. In addition, interventions, such as spinal immobilization, which would have been performed immediately in some cases, were not shown in the video to give you the opportunity to make all the decisions about patient care once the video concludes.

The video controls are similar to those found in many popular media players. Here is what each one does:

II PAUSE—Pauses or "freezes" the video on the current frame.

▶ PLAY—Resumes playing the video from the point where it has been paused or from the beginning if the video has been stopped.

■ STOP—Stops the video entirely. To restart the video, you must click **PLAY** (**▶**).

◀◀ REWIND—Restarts the video from the beginning.

▶▶ FORWARD—Jumps several frames forward in the video.

Two slider bars are also provided. The long slider bar across most of the width of the screen allows you to scroll back and forth to any point in the video. Simply click and hold the triangle (▲), then drag it to the left to go to an earlier moment or to the right to go to a later moment. The short slider bar on the far right controls the volume of the video's audio. A mute button between the two slider bars can be clicked to turn off the audio altogether.

When the video reaches the end, it automatically will forward you to the patient care interface, which is described below. If you want to skip the video altogether and go directly to the patient care interface, you can click on the **PROCEED** button at the bottom of the video screen.

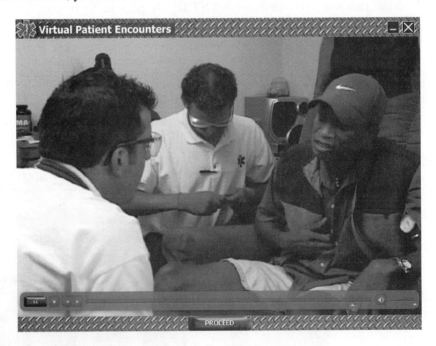

PATIENT CARE INTERFACE

The patient care interface consists of three panels: (1) Patient Care Panel, (2) Patient Visual Panel, and (3) Running Log as described in the following text.

Patient Care Panel

The Patient Care Panel runs along the left side of the screen and consists primarily of two distinct areas (shown at the top of the following page): (1) contains all the controls for performing assessments and (2) contains all the controls for performing interventions.

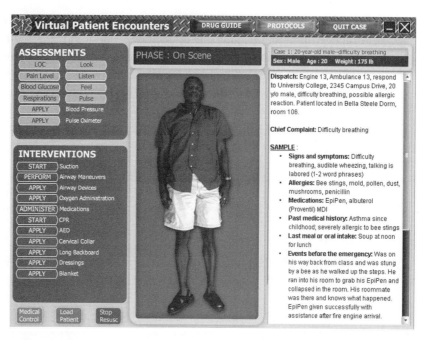

Assessment Controls

The assessment controls allow you to gather information on each patient so you can decide which interventions would be appropriate to care for him or her. These control buttons allow you to perform your patient assessments. Each button is described individually.

LOC (Level of Consciousness)—Click the **LOC** button to reveal the patient's current level of consciousness in the running log on the right side of the screen. In some cases the patient's orientation will be displayed below the level of consciousness if it is pertinent to the case. Be aware that the patient's level of consciousness may change, depending on what interventions you perform.

Pain Level—Click the **Pain Level** button to reveal the patient's current pain level on the 1-to-10 scale. The patient's pain level can increase or decrease, depending on your treatment.

Blood Glucose—Click the **Blood Glucose** button to reveal the patient's current blood glucose reading.

Respirations—Click the **Respirations** button to reveal the patient's current respiratory rate and quality. The respiration rate and quality can also be affected by your patient care decisions.

Pulse—Click the **Pulse** button to reveal the patient's current pulse rate, regularity, and strength. Your patient care decisions can affect these three measurements.

Blood Pressure—Click the **APPLY** button for blood pressure to place a blood pressure cuff on the patient and to receive your first reading. Once the cuff is on the patient, you only need to click the **READ** button that appears to the right for subsequent readings. If you want to remove the blood pressure cuff, you can click the **REMOVE** button that replaces the **APPLY** button.

Pulse Oximeter—Click the **APPLY** button for pulse oximeter to place a finger clip on the patient and to receive your first oxygen saturation (SaO_2) reading. Once the clip is on the patient, you only need to click the **READ** button that appears to the right for subsequent readings. If you want to remove the finger clip, you can click the **REMOVE** button that replaces the **APPLY** button. Interventions such as administering oxygen to the patient in respiratory distress can affect SaO_2 readings.

Look—Click the **Look** button to open a "wizard" that allows you to receive visual information about the patient's head and neck, chest and abdomen, upper extremities, lower extremities, back, and genitalia. Simply click on the body area you want to know about, and then click **ASSESS**. (Click **CANCEL** if you want to exit the wizard.) The following information is displayed in the running log for each body area:

Head and Neck
- Pupil size*
- Pupil reactivity*
- Skin color*
- Mouth*
- Nose*
- Other observations
- DCAP-BTLS

Chest and Abdomen
- Chest excursion*
- Skin color*
- Other observations
- DCAP-BTLS

Upper Extremities
- Skin color*
- Other observations
- DCAP-BTLS

Lower Extremities
- Skin color*
- Other observations
- DCAP-BTLS

Back
- Skin color*
- Other observations
- DCAP-BTLS

Genitalia
- Other observations
- DCAP-BTLS

The above items with an asterisk may change in response to your treatment decisions; do not forget to reassess often.

Listen—Click the **Listen** button to open a wizard that allows you to receive aural information about the patient's heart and lungs. Simply click on the organ you want to know about, and then click **ASSESS**. (Click **CANCEL** if you want to exit the wizard.) The following information is displayed in the running log for each:

Heart
- Heart rate*
- Heart regularity*

Lungs
- Left lung sounds*
- Right lung sounds*

The above items with an asterisk may change in response to your treatment decisions; do not forget to reassess often.

Feel—Click the **Feel** button to open a wizard that allows you to receive tactile information about the patient's head and neck, chest and abdomen, upper extremities, lower extremities, and back. Simply click on the body area you want to know about and then click **ASSESS**. (Click **CANCEL** if you want to exit the wizard.) The following information is displayed in the running log for each body area:

Head and Neck
- Skin temperature*
- Skin moisture*
- Other observations
- DCAP-BTLS

Chest and Abdomen
- Skin temperature*
- Skin moisture*
- Other observations
- DCAP-BTLS

Upper Extremities
- Skin temperature*
- Skin moisture*
- Other observations
- DCAP-BTLS

Lower Extremities
- Skin temperature*
- Skin moisture*
- Other observations
- DCAP-BTLS

Back
- Skin temperature*
- Skin moisture*
- Other observations
- DCAP-BTLS

The above items with an asterisk may change in response to your treatment decisions; do not forget to reassess often.

Intervention Controls

The intervention buttons will allow you to treat each patient in accordance with what you have learned in your textbook and in class, as well as what you think are the issues with each patient based on information you have gathered from the opening video, the patient's history, and any assessments you have performed. Each intervention that you perform may cause realistic changes in the patient, which you can determine by conducting ongoing assessments. Each intervention button is described individually below.

Suction—Click **START** to clear the patient's airway. Click **STOP** to end suctioning.

Airway Maneuvers—Click **PERFORM** to open a wizard that will allow you to choose to perform an abdominal thrust, a head-tilt/chin-lift, or a jaw thrust. Simply click on the maneuver you would like to perform.

Airway Devices—Click **APPLY** to open a wizard that will allow you to choose from the following airway devices:

- Oropharyngeal airway
- Nasopharyngeal airway

Click **REMOVE** to remove the airway device currently in use.

Oxygen Administration—Click **APPLY** to open a wizard that will allow you select from the following types of oxygen and ventilation devices:

- Nasal cannula
- Nonrebreather mask
- Bag-mask at 12 breaths/min
- Bag-mask at 20 breaths/min

Once you select one of the above devices, you will be prompted to select an oxygen flow rate. Click **REMOVE** to remove the type of oxygen or ventilation device currently in use.

Medications—Click **ADMINISTER** to open a wizard that allows you to administer medications to the patient.

The wizard has four steps:

1. Select the medication you want to administer from the list of generic drug names displayed (see figure below). Please note that when a patient has physician-prescribed medications, they will appear in the list in addition to the medications you can administer as an EMT. If you want to look up more information about a drug, click the **Drug Guide** button. This button will open a searchable resource that will be described in greater detail later in this orientation session. Highlight the medication you want to administer by clicking on its name, and then click **NEXT**. (Click **CANCEL** to exit the wizard altogether.)

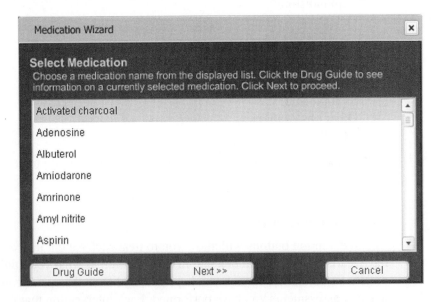

2. Select the route you want to use to administer the drug you selected in the first step. You can review the list of routes using the scroll bar on the right. Highlight the route you want to use, and then click **NEXT**. (Click **CANCEL** to exit the wizard altogether.) If you select an incorrect route for the drug you selected at the first step, you will receive a message to that effect and be instructed to click **BACK** and make a different route selection. Be aware that your incorrect route selection will be recorded on the running log, so make your selections carefully.

3. Select the dose you want to administer of the drug you selected in the first step. Be aware that each dose may have a different effect on the patient. Highlight the dose you want to administer, and then click **NEXT**. (Click **CANCEL** to exit the wizard altogether.)

4. The last step allows you to confirm all your selections before committing to them. Read over what you selected; if all selections are what you want, then click **FINISH**. If you want to make modifications, click **BACK** to return to the step where you want to make changes. Make your changes, and click **NEXT** until you get back to the confirmation step. As always, **CANCEL** will close the wizard without any effect on the patient.

CPR—Click **START** to begin performing cardiopulmonary resuscitation (CPR) on the patient. Click **STOP** to stop CPR.

AED—Click **APPLY** to place the defibrillator pads of an automated external defibrillator (AED) on the patient. Click **REMOVE** to remove the pads. To defibrillate the patient, click on the **SHOCK** button that appears in the panel to the right. This selection will open a wizard. Click **ANALYZE** first to determine whether a shock is advised in a message that appears in the running log. If advised, click **SHOCK**, and a shock will be delivered to the patient. If not advised, clicking **SHOCK** will not deliver a shock to the patient; however, the fact that you tried to do so will be recorded in the running log. You can click **CANCEL** to close the wizard without any effects on the patient.

Cervical Collar—Click **APPLY** to place a cervical collar on the patient. Click **REMOVE** to remove it.

Long Backboard—Click **APPLY** to place the patient on a long backboard. Click **REMOVE** to remove it.

Dressings—Click **APPLY** to place dressings on any wounds the patient may have. (Nothing will happen if the patient does not have wounds.) Click **REMOVE** to remove the dressings.

Blanket—Click **APPLY** to place a blanket on the patient. Click **REMOVE** to remove the blanket.

"Other" Buttons

Three additional buttons below the intervention controls level are available for use during patient care:

Medical Direction—Click the **Medical Direction** button if you want to contact medical direction. In this program you can contact medical direction to request additional orders or to request permission to stop resuscitation. Consult medical direction if you are having trouble figuring out which protocol(s) to follow for a particular case. They will eventually point you in the right direction. They will give you permission to stop resuscitation only if resuscitating the patient is not possible.

Stop Resusc—If medical direction gives you permission to stop resuscitation, you may click the **Stop Resusc** button. If you click the **Stop Resusc** button, you will be asked to confirm your decision. If you click *yes* to confirm, stopping resuscitation will be recorded in your log. Keep in mind that if you stop resuscitation without requesting permission from medical direction or if permission was denied, all of this will be recorded in your log for your instructor to evaluate.

Load/Unload Patient—When you first enter the patient care interface, you are considered to be "on scene." While on scene this button will display as **Load Patient**. Click this button when you believe transporting the patient is most appropriate. Your decision to load will be recorded in the running log in the context of all your assessments and interventions. Once you have loaded the patient, you are considered to be in transit and this button changes to display as **Unload Patient**.

You may have noticed that time is not counted in this program. Although this is a luxury you will not have in real life, removing the time element allows you to think about your decisions before you make them, rather than simply trying to "beat the clock," particularly because assessments and interventions are not done in real time. *Virtual Patient Encounters* is not intended to be used as a game.

Although the study guide may pose situations in which you have limited time in transit and asks questions about how you would adjust your treatment, in the software program you can continue performing interventions and assessments while in transit for as long as you believe you can make a difference. Once there is nothing more you can do besides provide support and monitor your patient, then you can click **UNLOAD PATIENT**.

Patient Visual Panel

The panel in the middle of the interface displays the patient in the supine position from a top-down perspective (shown below).

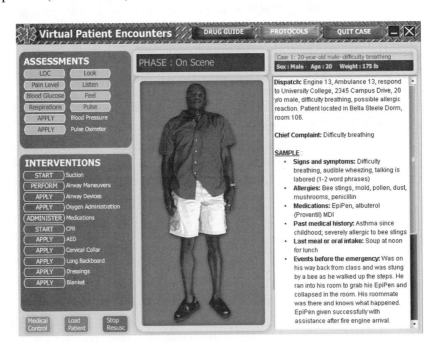

As you perform your assessments and interventions, the equipment you use appears on the patient in this panel. For example, when you click **APPLY Blood Pressure**, a blood pressure cuff will appear on the patient's arm; and when you click **APPLY Oxygen Administration** and select a nonrebreather mask, an image of a nonrebreather mask will appear on the patient; and so on. The patient visual panel is intended to give you a visual indication of what equipment is currently in use on the patient. The equipment images are representative of real equipment but may not always appear exactly as they would in real life; for example, when a long backboard is used, the patient would be secured to it with straps and a head immobilization device.

When you start CPR using the intervention buttons, you will see a pair of hands repeatedly compressing the patient's chest. These hands will give you a visual indication that CPR is in progress. When you stop CPR, the hands will disappear.

The patient is supine to best display the equipment that is in use. This position does not represent the position in which the patient is found nor does it necessarily represent the position in which you would place the patient to perform proper care. Questions about positioning of each of the patients will be found in the study guide lessons.

Above the patient visual, a display indicates whether you are "On Scene" or "In Transit."

Running Log

The running log is seen on the right side of the interface (shown below).

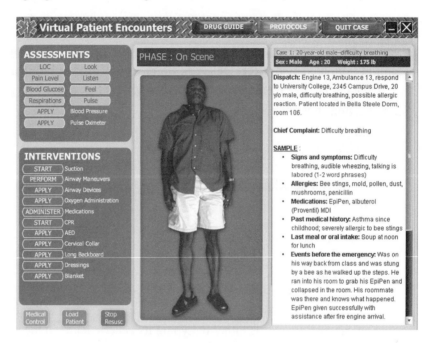

When you first enter the patient care interface after watching the video, the log will display the initial dispatch that you heard, as well as the patient's chief complaint and history in SAMPLE/OPQRST format. You should read this information before making any assessment or intervention decisions because doing so will provide a more complete picture than the video alone.

Once you begin making assessments, the data and observations appear in the running log in the order that you perform the assessments below the **Now On Scene** heading. This running log lets you know what is happening with the patient and, by reassessing, what is changing about the patient.

All interventions that you perform are also recorded in the running log. Interventions are always listed in italics to distinguish them from assessments. All the choices you make within the steps of the intervention wizards are recorded on the log; for example, when administering medications, the dose and the route are recorded in addition to the drug name.

Certain messages appear in the log in red type, either to notify you that something drastic has changed about your patient or to let you know that something you tried to do was not possible and why. For example, if your patient becomes unconscious while you are treating him or her, you may receive the message, "Your patient's condition has changed. You need to reassess," or "Patient is exhibiting seizure activity." If you were to try to insert an airway device while administering oxygen, you would receive a message such as, "Unable to perform oropharyngeal airway, breathing apparatus already in place." Once you remove the breathing apparatus, you can insert the airway device.

As your running log fills up with more and more information, you can use the scroll bar on the right to scroll up and down, perhaps to compare assessment data before and after a particular intervention.

Note that the case number and complaint, as well as the patient's gender, age, and weight, are listed for your information across the top of the running log.

REFERENCE RESOURCES

Across the top of the interface, you will see a blue button marked **DRUG GUIDE** and a yellow button labeled **PROTOCOLS**, which can be used as reference resources.

Clicking **DRUG GUIDE** will open a new window in which you can review the following information about medications:

- Class
- Trade names
- Description
- Onset and duration
- Indications
- Contraindications
- Adverse reactions
- Drug interactions
- How supplied
- Dosage and administration
- Special considerations

You can look up a drug either by typing its generic name in the search field at the top of the window or by scrolling through the list on the left and clicking directly on its name. To close the drug guide window, click on the **X** in the upper right corner.

Clicking **PROTOCOLS** opens a different window that displays a menu of 23 protocols. One or more of these protocols will be appropriate for each of the 15 cases found in this program. Simply click on the name of the protocol you want to open. Note that each protocol is divided into sections by scope of practice. Although the protocols will not tell you exactly what to do, keep in mind that they should put you on the right track if you have selected protocols that are relevant to the patient you are treating.

To return to the listing of protocols, click on **Return to List**. To close the protocols window, click on the **X** in the upper right corner.

SUMMARY MENU

Three ways are provided to navigate to the summary menu, two of which you already know about; that is, by clicking **Unload Patient** while in transit or by clicking **Stop Resusc** after you have been given permission to do so by medical direction. The third way is by clicking the red **QUIT CASE** button to the right of the **PROTOCOLS** button. Use this button to leave a case when you want to skip it or to switch to another case. Many study guide lessons may only require you to watch the video and read the history before answering the questions, in which case you will be directed to simply quit the case.

The summary menu itself offers four choices as described below:

LOG—Click the **Log** button to view, save, or print the log from the case you just completed. The information that was recorded in the running log during patient care is now displayed full screen for you to review easily (shown below).

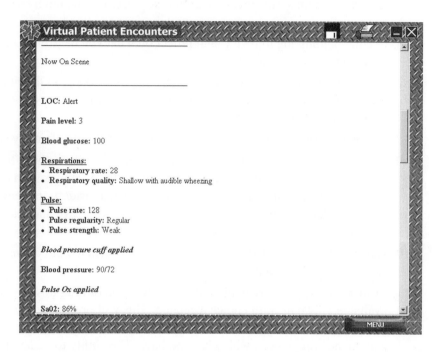

All of the summative lessons will instruct you to review the log of your patient care while answering questions in the study guide. Click the icon of the floppy disk in the upper right corner to save your log as a rich text file, or click the icon of a printer to print out a hard copy. Be prepared for your instructor to ask you to submit your logs for his or her evaluation. Click **MENU** in the lower right corner to return to the summary menu.

RESTART—Click the **Restart** button to return to the patient selection screen. Be aware that unless you printed or saved a copy of your log from the case you just completed, a record of what you did will not be available to retrieve.

CREDITS—Click the **Credits** button to display a listing of all the people and organizations that contributed to the development of the simulation software. Click **RETURN TO MENU** to return to the summary menu.

EXIT—Click the **Exit** button to close the entire *Virtual Patient Encounters* program. As with clicking **RESTART**, be aware that unless you printed or saved a copy of your log from the case you just completed, no record of what you did will be available to retrieve.

TIPS FOR USING *VIRTUAL PATIENT ENCOUNTERS*

Last, the following tips will improve your experience with *Virtual Patient Encounters* and can enhance your knowledge and prepare you for facing the uncertainty of the streets.

1. Always read the assigned chapter(s) before attempting the study guide lessons.
2. Keep your textbook handy as a reference while you work through the lessons.
3. Take your time—things in the program are not happening in real time. Reflect on your next action before you perform it.

4. Be sure to think about the appropriate sequence of actions. In real life, many assessments and interventions will happen simultaneously. When working in this program, you have to perform things one step at a time.

5. Do not assume that others are performing certain skills or assessments as they would on a real call. You must specifically identify each assessment and intervention to be performed on the call.

6. Use the running log to review and reflect on what you have done so you can choose your next intervention or assessment.

7. Watch for the key messages (in red type) that may appear in the running log to indicate that the patient's condition has changed drastically. Failure to see one of these messages can lead you down the wrong path.

8. Just as you would in real life, reassess often, particularly after any significant intervention.

9. Because you do not interact with a live patient, you will not have the benefit of the information and clues that you would normally have. Things such as how the patient feels (except for pain scale), his or her body language, and additional environmental clues will not be available. Simply use the information that you have and make the best judgments you can, based on the information you are given.

10. When you use the software program, follow the bulleted directions provided in the lessons and answer the relevant questions.

11. In some cases, you may think that an intervention or drug dose is appropriate but not available. Make the best choice available. This will prepare you for the "real world" of EMS where everything you need is also not available. Sometimes you have to improvise and do the best you can with what you have. The ability to make the most with the least is often what makes a great EMT.

12. As previously mentioned, the protocols follow the guidelines in your textbook—sometimes these will vary from your local protocols. Discuss any variations and the reasons for them with your instructor.

13. The exact nature of illness or injury may not be perfectly clear in all cases. In other cases, you may have a pretty clear clinical impression, but you might not have any interventions that can correct the patient's problem. This scenario also mirrors real EMS practice. Simply perform the best interventions at your disposal and transport the patient when appropriate. Limitations in the prehospital setting will always occur.

We hope that *Virtual Patient Encounters* will be just one more tool to build your knowledge and improve your critical thinking ability as you move toward your goal of becoming an EMT. Best wishes and good luck!

Introduction to Emergency Medical Care

Reading Assignment: Read Chapter 1, Introduction to Emergency Medical Care, in *EMT Prehospital Care,* Fourth Edition.

Case 10: 25-year-old female—abdominal pain

Objectives:

On completion of this lesson, the student will be able to perform the following:

- Describe how the positive attributes of the professional emergency medical technician (EMT) are demonstrated during patient care activities.

- Outline the role of medical direction on this call.

EXERCISE 1

 CD-ROM Activity

 Time: 15 minutes

- Sign into the software by entering your name in the name tag and clicking **Enter**.
- Choose the case by clicking on ***Case 10: 25-year-old female—abdominal pain***.
- Listen to the dispatch, or read it in the right panel (or both).
- Click **Start**, and watch the entire video. Once the video has concluded, you are "on scene."
- Read the history log on the right side of the screen.

1. Describe specific behaviors you observed of the EMTs on this call that demonstrate the attributes of the professional EMT. If the attribute is not seen on this call, write "not observed."

Attribute	Specific Behavior Observed on This Call
Sensitive awareness of the environment and those around them	
Personal behavior (attitude)	

Attribute	Specific Behavior Observed on This Call
Self-composure	
Professional appearance	
Maintenance of knowledge and skills	

2. On this case, why will it be important for the EMT to have a good working knowledge of hospital designation and categorization?

3. Describe what type of direct (online) or indirect (medical oversight) medical direction the EMTs may need on this call.

     a. Online:

     b. Offline (medical oversight):

➡   • Click **Quit Case**, and you will be taken to the summary menu.
     • Click **Exit** to close the program, or **Restart** to continue with another lesson.

Well-Being of the EMT

∞ **Reading Assignment:** Read Chapter 2, Well-Being of the EMT, in *EMT Prehospital Care, Fourth Edition.*

Case 3: 7-year-old female—seizure

Case 13: 5-month-old-male—unresponsive

Objectives:

On completion of this lesson, the student will be able to perform the following:

- Discuss measures that can be taken to reduce the incidence of injury or illness on an emergency medical services (EMS) call.
- Recognize normal responses to death and dying.
- Identify wellness practices that minimize the risk of injury on the job.

EXERCISE 1

 CD-ROM Activity

 Time: 15 minutes

- Sign into the software by entering your name in the name tag and clicking **Enter**.
- Choose the case by clicking on *Case 13: 5-month-old male—unresponsive*.
- Listen to the dispatch, or read it in the right panel (or both).
- Click **Start**, and watch the entire video. Once the video has concluded, you are "on scene."
- Read the history log on the right side of the screen.

1. What stressors will you face on this call?

2. Match the following statements that a parent whose child is dying may make to the stage of grief from Table 2-6, Stages of Grief, that the statement represents.

Statement	Stage of Grief
"Hurry, you're not doing anything to help him. Don't you care?"	
"If he's okay, I swear I'll never put him down to sleep on his stomach again."	
"He's dead. I just know it."	
"He'll be fine. I think he just passed out. They'll make him all better."	
"I'll never survive this. I can't take it. I won't live without him."	

3. What measures were the EMTs using to reduce their risk of exposure to blood or bloody body fluids? Discuss why you feel these measures are adequate or not adequate.

4. List at least five behaviors that might indicate that your partner is experiencing severe stress in the first few days after this call.

5. What steps can you take to deal with any strong feelings you may have after this call is over?

 • Click **Quit Case**, and you will be taken to the summary menu.

EXERCISE 2

 CD-ROM Activity

 Time: 15 minutes

 • Click **Restart** from the summary menu.
   • Choose the case by clicking on *Case 3: 7-year-old female—seizure*.
   • Listen to the dispatch, or read it in the right panel (or both).
   • Click **Start**, and watch the entire video. Once the video has concluded, you are "on scene."
   • Read the history log on the right side of the screen.

The crew suspects that this child has bacterial meningitis because of her signs and symptoms and her rash.

6. Describe measures that the crew should take after the call to minimize their risk of becoming infected with a contagious disease.

7. How should the crew clean the ambulance if tests confirm that this patient has bacterial meningitis?

8. What steps should all EMS providers take during and before going on calls to minimize the risk of getting an infectious disease on the job?

→   • Click **Quit Case**, and you will be taken to the summary menu.
     • Click **Exit** to close the program, or **Restart** to continue with another lesson.

Medicolegal and Ethical Issues

Reading Assignment: Read Chapter 3, Medicolegal and Ethical Issues, in *EMT Prehospital Care,* Fourth Edition.

Case 8: 38-year-old male—suicide attempt

Objectives:

On completion of this lesson, the student will be able to perform the following:

- Relate the legal principles of assault and battery to the restraint issue in this case.
- Discuss how consent is obtained during care of the patient in this case.
- Apply the elements of negligence to a variation of this case.

EXERCISE 1

  CD-ROM Activity

  Time: 20 minutes

- Sign into the software by entering your name in the name tag and clicking **Enter**.
- Choose the case by clicking on *Case 8: 38-year-old male—suicide attempt*.
- Listen to the dispatch, or read it in the right panel (or both).
- Click **Start**, and watch the entire video. Once the video has concluded, you are "on scene."
- Read the history log on the right side of the screen.

1. Was it appropriate for the EMTs to restrain and transport this patient against his will? Explain your answer.

2. Research the involuntary admission laws in your state. How long can this patient be held against his will? Who has the authority to hold him for longer than the initial phase?

3. What type of consent applies in this case?

4. Should you ask the patient about his wishes for care and transport?

5. You fail to assess the restrained patient and he vomits, aspirates, and dies. List the four elements needed to prove negligence, and explain how the plaintiff's attorney would have been able to prove them in this case to satisfy the claim.

Element	Why the Claim Is Satisfied or Not Satisfied

 • Click **Quit Case** and you will be taken to the summary menu.
• Click **Exit** to close the program, or **Restart** to continue with another lesson.

The Human Body

/OZO **Reading Assignment:** Read Chapter 4, The Human Body, in *EMT Prehospital Care,* Fourth Edition.

Case 11: 32-year-old male—gunshot wounds

Objectives:

On completion of this lesson, the student will be able to perform the following:

• Use directional terms appropriately to describe wound locations.

• Relate the injuries observed to the anatomic structures involved.

• Describe alterations in body function that should be anticipated based on the wounds observed.

EXERCISE 1

 CD-ROM Activity

 Time: 10 minutes

→ • Sign into the software by entering your name in the name tag and clicking **Enter**.
• Choose the case by clicking on *Case 11: 32-year-old male—gunshot wounds*.
• Listen to the dispatch, or read it in the right panel (or both).
• Click **Start**, and watch the entire video. Once the video has concluded, you are "on scene."
• Read the history log on the right side of the screen.

1. Describe the location of the injuries using proper anatomic terminology.

   a. The neck wound was located _____ to the midline of the neck.

   b. The chest wound was located _____ to the nipple and

   _____ to the clavicle.

   c. The abdominal wound was located _____ and

   _____ to the umbilicus. The abdominal wound was

   located in the _____ quadrant of the abdomen.

   d. The patient was found in the _____ position.

2. Predict which anatomic structures are located beneath each wound.
   a. Neck wound:

   b. Chest wound:

c. Abdominal wound:

3. Predict alterations in the normal physiology of body systems that may be affected by these wounds:

a. Neck wound:

b. Chest wound:

c. Abdominal wound:

4. If the gunshot wound was located on the left side of the abdomen, predict the organs that might be injured.

→ • Click **Quit Case** and you will be taken to the summary menu.
   • Click **Exit** to close the program, or **Restart** to continue with another lesson.

Lifting and Moving Patients

Reading Assignment: Read Chapter 5, Lifting and Moving Patients, in *EMT Prehospital Care,* Fourth Edition.

Case 1: 20-year-old male—difficulty breathing

Case 12: 57-year-old male—man down

Objectives:

On completion of this lesson, the student will be able to perform the following:

- Identify appropriate lifting techniques.
- Describe body mechanics that promote safe lifting.
- Given a scenario, select the appropriate device for lifting and moving a patient.
- Describe the appropriate patient position for transport.

EXERCISE 1

 CD-ROM Activity

 Time: 10 minutes

- Sign into the software by entering your name in the name tag and clicking **Enter**.
- Choose the case by clicking on *Case 12: 57-year-old male—man down*.
- Listen to the dispatch, or read it in the right panel (or both).
- Click **Start**, and watch the entire video. Once the video has concluded, you are "on scene."
- Read the history log on the right side of the screen.

1. What lifting techniques did you observe the emergency medical technician (EMT) demonstrate that should reduce the risk of back injury on the job? How could he improve his lifting technique?

2. If this patient is unable to sit up to move to the stretcher, describe how the EMTs will move him to the stretcher.

3. How should this patient be positioned on the stretcher? Explain your answer.

- Click **Quit Case** and you will be taken to the summary menu.

EXERCISE 2

 CD-ROM Activity

 Time: 10 minutes

- Click **Restart** from the summary menu.
- Choose the case by clicking on *Case 1: 20-year-old male—difficulty breathing*.
- Listen to the dispatch, or read it in the right panel (or both).
- Click **Start**, and watch the entire video. Once the video has concluded, you are "on scene."
- Read the history log on the right side of the screen.

4. List measures you can take to minimize the risk of injury to the crew or the patient if this patient is conscious but cannot walk down the stairs.

5. What individual characteristics about the EMTs did you note that might reduce their risk of injury or illness?

6. How will you position this patient on the stretcher? Explain your answer.

- Click **Quit Case**, and you will be taken to the summary menu.
- Click **Exit** to close the program, or **Restart** to continue with another lesson.

Airway

∞ **Reading Assignment:** Read Chapter 6, Airway, in *EMT Prehospital Care,* Fourth Edition.

Case 1: 20-year-old male—difficulty breathing

Case 2: 56-year-old female—fell

Case 5: 40-year-old male—vomiting blood

Case 6: 16-year-old female—unknown medical

Objectives:

On completion of this lesson, the student will be able to perform the following:

- Describe assessment of airway, ventilation, and oxygenation.
- List factors that may impair normal oxygenation.
- Identify measures to improve oxygenation and ventilation.

EXERCISE 1

 Preparation Activity

 Time: 10 minutes

Before beginning the simulation, answer the following questions.

   1. What conditions or diseases might reduce oxygen levels in the blood?

   2. List some ways a patient might be treated for low oxygen levels.

   3. What conditions or diseases impair circulation of red blood cells to the tissue?

EXERCISE 2

 CD-ROM Activity

 Time: 10 minutes

 • Sign into the software by entering your name in the name tag and clicking **Enter**.
     • Choose the case by clicking on *Case 1: 20-year-old male—difficulty breathing*.
     • Listen to the dispatch, or read it in the right panel (or both).
     • Click **Start**, and watch the entire video. Once the video has concluded, you are "on scene."
     • Read the history log on the right side of the screen.
     • Perform your initial assessment using the **Assessment** buttons in the left panel.

   4. What is causing James's difficult breathing?

5. How would it benefit James if oxygen was applied?

6. Did pulse oximetry provide useful information in this case? Why?

 • Click **Quit Case**, and you will be taken to the summary menu.
• Click on **Log**.
• To save your log, click the disk icon. To print your log, click the printer icon.
• Click **Menu** to return to the summary menu.

EXERCISE 3

 CD-ROM Activity

 Time: 10 minutes

 • Click **Restart** from the summary menu.
• Choose the case by clicking on *Case 2: 56-year-old female—fell*.
• Listen to the dispatch, or read it in the right panel (or both).
• Click **Start**, and watch the entire video. Once the video has concluded, you are "on scene."
• Read the history log on the right side of the screen.
• Perform your initial assessment using the **Assessment** buttons in the left panel.

7. List the signs of respiratory distress you observe in this patient.

8. The original dispatch was for a woman who fell. List possible causes of her dyspnea.

9. What may make management of this patient's airway, oxygenation, and ventilation more difficult?

10. Did pulse oximetry provide valuable information in this patient? Why?

 • Click **Quit Case**, and you will be taken to the summary menu.
   • Click on **Log**.
   • To save your log, click the disk icon. To print your log, click the printer icon.
   • Click **Menu** to return to the summary menu.

EXERCISE 4

 CD-ROM Activity

 Time: 10 minutes

→ • Click **Restart** from the summary menu.
   • Choose the case by clicking on *Case 5: 40-year-old male—vomiting blood*.
   • Listen to the dispatch, or read it in the right panel (or both).

11. Before beginning the video, review the steps for suctioning and list them.

→ • Click **Start**, and watch the entire video. Once the video has concluded, you are "on scene."
   • Read the history log on the right side of the screen.
   • Perform your initial assessment using the **Assessment** buttons in the left panel.

12. What concerns do you have about this patient's airway?

13. How would you prepare yourself to care for this patient's airway?

14. Did pulse oximetry provide useful information in this case? Why?

→ • Click **Quit Case**, and you will be taken to the summary menu.
   • Click on **Log**.
   • To save your log, click the disk icon. To print your log, click the printer icon.
   • Click **Menu** to return to the summary menu.

EXERCISE 5

 CD-ROM Activity

 Time: 10 minutes

 • Click **Restart** from the summary menu.
 • Choose the case by clicking on *Case 6: 16-year-old female—unknown medical*.
 • Listen to the dispatch, or read it in the right panel (or both).

15. Before beginning the video, review the steps for insertion of a nasopharyngeal airway and list them.

 • Click **Start**, and watch the entire video. Once the video has concluded, you are "on scene."
 • Read the history log on the right side of the screen.
 • Perform your initial assessment using the **Assessment** buttons in the left panel.

16. What are your management priorities for Sarah?

17. Did pulse oximetry provide valuable information about Sarah? Why?

 • Click **Quit Case** and you will be taken to the summary menu.
 • Click on **Log**.
 • To save your log, click the disk icon. To print your log, click the printer icon.
 • Click **Exit** to close the program, or **Restart** to continue with another lesson.

LESSON 7

Patient Assessment

👓 **Reading Assignment:** Read Chapter 7, Patient Assessment, in *EMT Prehospital Care,* Fourth Edition.

Case 1: 20-year-old male—difficulty breathing
Case 2: 56-year-old female—fell
Case 3: 7-year-old female—seizure
Case 5: 40-year-old male—vomiting blood
Case 6: 16-year-old female—unknown medical
Case 7: 8-year-old male—submersion
Case 8: 38-year-old male—suicide attempt
Case 9: 22-year-old female—assault
Case 10: 25-year-old female—abdominal pain
Case 11: 32-year-old male—gunshot wounds
Case 12: 57-year-old male—man down

Objectives:

On completion of this lesson, the student will be able to perform the following:

• Outline the elements of the scene size-up.
• Recognize potential hazards on an emergency scene.
• Recall the components of initial (primary) assessment.
• Identify the essential primary assessment information from the scenario.
• Recognize abnormal assessment findings when given a patient scenario.
• Outline the technique of vital sign assessment.
• Describe the significance of the SAMPLE history.
• Identify situations in which a rapid trauma assessment would be appropriate.
• Explain the value of reassessment.
• Discuss how to apply the phases of the patient assessment to each patient situation.

27

EXERCISE 1

 CD-ROM Activity

 Time: 20 minutes

- Sign into the software by entering your name in the name tag and clicking **Enter**.
- Choose the case by clicking on *Case 2: 56-year-old female—fell*.
- Listen to the dispatch, or read it in the right panel (or both).
- Click **Start**, and watch the entire video. Once the video has concluded, you are "on scene."

1. List each component of the scene size-up, and describe your assessment of each component on this case.

Scene Size-Up Component	Assessment

2. What is your general impression of this patient?

3. What difficulties did the EMTs encounter in obtaining this patient's medical history?

4. How can they overcome some of these difficulties?

- Read the history log on the right side of the screen.

5. What additional assessments will be needed for this patient?

6. List at least three possible causes of the signs and symptoms you have gathered up to this point for this case.

➡ • Click **Quit Case**, and you will be taken to the summary menu.

EXERCISE 2

 CD-ROM Activity

 Time: 15 minutes

- Click **Restart** from the summary menu.
- Choose the case by clicking on *Case 3: 7-year-old female—seizure*.
- Listen to the dispatch, or read it in the right panel (or both).
- Click **Start**, and watch the entire video. Once the video has concluded, you are "on scene."
- Read the history log on the right side of the screen.

7. List the components of the scene size-up. Indicate your assessment of each component of the scene size-up on this case.

Scene Size-Up Component	Assessment

8. Do you have enough information to determine whether this case is related to illness or trauma? Explain your answer.

• Perform your initial assessment using the **Assessment** buttons in the left panel.

9. Based on the information you have from the primary assessment, how will you manage this child's airway and breathing?

10. What information did you gather from your initial inspection and palpation of the skin of this patient?

11. Obtain one initial set of vital signs for this case. Indicate any abnormal vital sign findings. Explain a possible reason for the abnormal vital sign findings based on the information you have obtained up to this point in the call.

Initial Vital Signs			Which Findings Are Abnormal?	Rationale for Any Abnormal Vital Sign Finding
BP	P	R		

12. Explain what priority you would assign this patient based on your initial assessment.

 • Click **Quit Case**, and you will be taken to the summary menu.

EXERCISE 3

 CD-ROM Activity

 Time: 15 minutes

 • Click **Restart** from the summary menu.
- Choose the case by clicking on *Case 5: 40-year-old male—vomiting blood*.
- Listen to the dispatch, or read it in the right panel (or both).
- Click **Start**, and watch the entire video. Once the video has concluded, you are "on scene."
- Read the history log on the right side of the screen.

13. List the components of the scene size-up. Indicate your assessment of each component of the scene size-up on this case.

Scene Size-Up Component	Assessment

Scene Size-Up Component	Assessment

14. What life threats do you expect to find in your initial assessment of this patient, based on the information from the scene size-up?

15. How should you assess this patient's airway?

16. If his airway is not patent, what measures should you anticipate having to use, based on the information you know to this point?

17. List the steps you will use to assess circulation during your primary assessment of this patient. What findings during the examination would indicate the patient is in shock?

Steps to Assess Circulation	Findings That Would Indicate Shock

- Perform your initial assessment using the **Assessment** buttons in the left panel.

18. Explain what priority you would assign this patient, based on your primary assessment.

19. Explain why you would or would not perform a detailed physical examination of this patient.

→ • Click **Quit Case**, and you will be taken to the summary menu.

EXERCISE 4

  CD-ROM Activity

 Time: 15 minutes

➡️ • Click **Restart** from the summary menu.
• Choose the case by clicking on *Case 1: 20-year-old male—difficulty breathing*.
• Listen to the dispatch, or read it in the right panel (or both).
• Click **Start**, and watch the entire video. Once the video has concluded, you are "on scene."
• Read the history log on the right side of the screen.

20. List the assessment priorities and information needed in the primary assessment of this patient.

21. Why is it important to listen carefully to the information provided by the emergency medical responders and campus person?

22. Using only the information you have from the initial dispatch and video information, identify the following:

   a. General impression of this patient

   b. His mental status

   c. His airway status

   d. His oxygenation and respiration status

   e. His circulatory status

23. Predict the life threats (if any) you will need to treat during the initial assessment of this patient. Explain your rationale.

24. List two possible causes of the symptoms presented in this case.

25. Based on the initial information you have at this point in the call, explain why you think this patient has either adequate or inadequate breathing when you arrive at the call.

26. What care should you provide for this patient's breathing, based on the information you have after the report by the first responders?

→ • Click **Quit Case**, and you will be taken to the summary menu.

EXERCISE 5

 CD-ROM Activity

 Time: 15 minutes

- Click **Restart** from the summary menu.
- Choose the case by clicking on *Case 6: 16-year-old female—unknown medical*.
- Listen to the dispatch, or read it in the right panel (or both).
- Click **Start**, and watch the entire video. Once the video has concluded, you are "on scene."
- Read the history log on the right side of the screen.

27. What interventions should you perform during the initial assessment, based on the information you have at present?

28. Based on the information you have that indicates that this patient has taken an overdose, what specific physical assessments will you perform that relate to this type of history?

29. What critical information did you obtain from the SAMPLE history that will affect her pre-hospital and in-hospital care?

Element	Findings	Significance	Possible Implications for Care
Signs and symptoms			

Element	Findings	Significance	Possible Implications for Care
Allergies			
Medicines			
Medical history			
Last meal/ menstrual period			
Events leading up to incident			

30. Because the patient is unconscious, what other resources will you need?

• Perform your initial assessment using the **Assessment** buttons in the left panel.

31. Describe your primary assessment findings is this patient.

Assessment Criteria	This Patient
General impression	
Mental status	
Airway	
Breathing	
Circulation	

32. What priority should be assigned to this patient? Explain your answer.

33. After you complete your initial examination and treatment of this patient, explain what you should assess during the ongoing assessment while you transport her and how often you should perform your ongoing assessment.

 • Click **Quit Case**, and you will be taken to the summary menu.

EXERCISE 6

 CD-ROM Activity

 Time: 15 minutes

 • Click **Restart** from the summary menu.
- Choose the case by clicking on *Case 12: 57-year-old male—man down*.
- Listen to the dispatch, or read it in the right panel (or both).
- Click **Start**, and watch the entire video. Once the video has concluded, you are "on scene."
- Read the history log on the right side of the screen.

34. What sources of information relative to the situation and the patient's condition did you have on this call?

35. What additional assessments should you perform on this patient?

36. What preliminary information do you have about his airway, breathing, and respiration status?

37. Describe how you will assess this patient's breathing status.

38. Explain whether capillary refill would or would not be a reliable assessment to perform on this patient.

39. List at least four possible causes of the symptoms presented in this case.

40. If you were to find the following vital signs during your primary assessment, explain whether they would be normal or abnormal for this patient and the significance of each finding.

Initial Assessment Finding	Normal or Abnormal Finding	Significance
Blood pressure: 70/50 mm Hg		
Pulse: 50 beats per minute		
Respirations: 6 per minute		

41. If you assessed the patient's blood pressure using a blood pressure cuff that covered one fourth of the diameter of his arm, would you expect his blood pressure reading to be higher than expected for his age, lower than expected for his age, or normal? Explain your answer.

42. When would you perform a detailed physical examination of this patient?

43. What would you be looking for when you perform a detailed physical examination of this patient?

44. On what specific body regions would you focus when performing the detailed physical examination of this patient? Explain your answer.

➡ • Click **Quit Case**, and you will be taken to the summary menu.

EXERCISE 7

 CD-ROM Activity

 Time: 15 minutes

- Click **Restart** from the summary menu.
- Choose the case by clicking on *Case 7: 8-year-old male—submersion*.
- Listen to the dispatch, or read it in the right panel (or both).
- Click **Start**, and watch the entire video. Once the video has concluded, you are "on scene."
- Read the history log on the right side of the screen.

45. What type of trauma assessment would you perform on this patient? Explain your answer.

- Perform your initial assessment using the **Assessment** buttons in the left panel.

46. List the components of the DCAPBTLS mnemonic, and record any findings identified on this call using this mnemonic.

	Component	Findings on This Call
D		
C		
A		
P		
B		
T		

	Component	Findings on This Call
L		
S		

 • Click **Quit Case**, and you will be taken to the summary menu.

EXERCISE 8

 CD-ROM Activity

 Time: 15 minutes

 • Click **Restart** from the summary menu.
- Choose the case by clicking on *Case 11: 32-year-old male—gunshot wounds*.
- Listen to the dispatch, or read it in the right panel (or both).
- Click **Start**, and watch the entire video. Once the video has concluded, you are "on scene."
- Read the history log on the right side of the screen.
- Perform your initial assessment using the **Assessment** buttons in the left panel.

47. Obtain one set of vital signs for this patient. Indicate any vital sign finding that is abnormal. Explain a possible reason for the abnormal vital sign finding, based on the information you have obtained up to this point on the call.

Initial Vital Signs			Which Findings Are Abnormal?	Rationale for Any Abnormal Vital Sign Finding
BP	P	R		

48. Identify other characteristics of the pulse you will evaluate while you are assessing the rate. Explain the significance of abnormal findings of these characteristics.

49. When you assess this patient's respirations, what should you assess other than the rate? Why are these additional assessments important?

50. What information did you gather from your initial inspection and palpation of the skin in this patient?

51. What specific findings will you look for during the rapid assessment of this patient?

    a. Neck

b. Chest

c. Abdomen

d. Back

52. Will you do a focused trauma assessment of any of this patient's injuries? Explain your answer.

 • Click **Quit Case**, and you will be taken to the summary menu.

EXERCISE 9

 CD-ROM Activity

 Time: 15 minutes

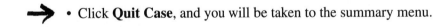 • Click **Restart** from the summary menu.
• Choose the case by clicking on ***Case 10: 25-year-old female—abdominal pain***.
• Listen to the dispatch, or read it in the right panel (or both).
• Click **Start**, and watch the entire video. Once the video has concluded, you are "on scene."
• Read the history log on the right side of the screen.

53. What communication barrier exists on this call? Explain how it may affect your assessment of this patient.

54. Does the presence of her translator during your assessment of the patient violate any HIPAA rules? Explain your answer.

55. What critical information did you obtain from the SAMPLE history that will affect her pre-hospital and in-hospital care?

Element	Findings	Significance	Possible Implications for Care
Signs and symptoms			
Allergies			
Medicines			

Element	Findings	Significance	Possible Implications for Care
Medical history			
Last meal/ menstrual period			
Events leading up to incident			

56. What specific findings will you look for when examining the following areas during the rapid assessment of this patient?

a. Abdomen:

b. Extremities:

c. Perineum:

➡ • Click **Quit Case**, and you will be taken to the summary menu.

EXERCISE 10

  CD-ROM Activity

 Time: 15 minutes

- Click **Restart** from the summary menu.
- Choose the case by clicking on *Case 7: 8-year-old male—submersion*.
- Listen to the dispatch, or read it in the right panel (or both).
- Click **Start**, and watch the entire video. Once the video has concluded, you are "on scene."
- Read the history log on the right side of the screen.

Assume that you are able to establish and maintain this patient's airway and breathing. You are en route to the hospital, and he is responsive only to painful stimuli.

57. Describe the specific findings you will look for as you perform the detailed examination of this patient in each body region listed, based on the history and mechanism of injury. List the potential injuries or problems that each of these findings may indicate.

Body Region	Specific Findings	Potential Injuries and Problems
Head		
Face		
Eyes		

Body Region	Specific Findings	Potential Injuries and Problems
Nose		
Mouth		
Neck		
Chest		
Abdomen		
Pelvis		
Arms and legs		

Body Region	Specific Findings	Potential Injuries and Problems
Back (performed while moving patient onto long spine board)		

  • Click **Quit Case**, and you will be taken to the summary menu.

EXERCISE 11

 CD-ROM Activity

 Time: 15 minutes

  • Click **Restart** from the summary menu.
• Choose the case by clicking on *Case 9: 22-year-old female—assault*.
• Listen to the dispatch, or read it in the right panel (or both).
• Click **Start**, and watch the entire video. Once the video has concluded, you are "on scene."
• Read the history log on the right side of the screen.

58. How will you perform the detailed physical examination of this patient's head and face?

59. Why is a detailed examination of this patient's head and face indicated?

60. Describe the order in which the detailed examination of this patient will be performed.

61. Will there be any body area you will NOT examine on this patient? Explain your answer.

→ • Click **Quit Case**, and you will be taken to the summary menu.

EXERCISE 12

 CD-ROM Activity

 Time: 15 minutes

 → • Click **Restart** from the summary menu.
  • Choose the case by clicking on *Case 8: 38-year-old male—suicide attempt*.
  • Listen to the dispatch, or read it in the right panel (or both).
  • Click **Start**, and watch the entire video. Once the video has concluded, you are "on scene."
  • Read the history log on the right side of the screen.
  • Perform your initial assessment using the **Assessment** buttons in the left panel.

62. This patient's initial vital signs did not indicate a critical life threat. How often should you reassess his vital signs?

63. What else should you reassess on this patient? Explain your rationale for each reassessment you would perform.

64. What intervention(s) would be indicated if you found the following when you reassessed the patient?

Reassessment Finding	Intervention
Heart rate: 30 bpm (beats per minute)	
Capillary refill in right hand: 6 seconds	
Oxygen saturation (SaO$_2$): 82%	
AVPU assessment: patient responds to painful stimulus	

Reassessment Finding	Intervention
Respiratory rate: 8 breaths per minute	
Blood pressure: 112/76 mm Hg	

- Click **Quit Case**, and you will be taken to the summary menu.
- Click **Exit** to close the program, or **Restart** to continue with another lesson.

Communications

⌒⌒ **Reading Assignment:** Read Chapter 8, Communications, in *EMT Prehospital Care*, Fourth Edition.

Case 2: 56-year-old female—fell
Case 9: 22-year-old female—assault
Case 10: 25-year-old female—abdominal pain

Objectives:

On completion of this lesson, the student will be able to perform the following:

- Identify therapeutic communication techniques used by the emergency medical technicians (EMTs) in selected cases.
- Recognize barriers to effective communication, and identify strategies that may be used to overcome them.
- Describe the importance of the dispatch information.
- Describe the effects of inadequate or inappropriate dispatch information.

EXERCISE 1

  CD-ROM Activity

 Time: 10 minutes

→
- Sign into the software by entering your name in the name tag and clicking **Enter**.
- Choose the case by clicking on *Case 2: 56-year-old female—fell*.
- Listen to the dispatch, or read it in the right panel (or both).
- Click **Start**, and watch the entire video. Once the video has concluded, you are "on scene."
- Read the history log on the right side of the screen.

1. Did the dispatch complaint relate directly to the patient's chief complaint?

2. Could the dispatch information in this case affect what equipment the EMTs bring into the patient's home? Explain your answer.

3. Did the EMTs focus on the dispatch information as the chief cause of illness? Explain your answer.

4. How could incorrect dispatch information delay the response to the scene?

5. After the EMT spoke with the patient's husband, what information should he communicate to his partner?

 • Click **Quit Case**, and you will be taken to the summary menu.

EXERCISE 2

 CD-ROM Activity

 Time: 15 minutes

• Click **Restart** from the summary menu.
• Choose the case by clicking on *Case 9: 22-year-old female—assault*.
• Listen to the dispatch, or read it in the right panel (or both).
• Click **Start**, and watch the entire video. Once the video has concluded, you are "on scene."
• Read the history log on the right side of the screen.

6. Describe the EMTs' communication with this patient as it relates to the following:

Communication Technique	EMTs on This Call
Develop contact with the patient	

Communication Technique	EMTs on This Call
Allow for a response	
Provide privacy	
Be professional	
Use effective body language	

7. What barriers to effective therapeutic communication existed on this call?

8. What strategies can EMTs use to overcome these barriers?

9. If the police officer had not been present, how might that have affected the interview?

 • Click **Quit Case**, and you will be taken to the summary menu.

EXERCISE 3

 CD-ROM Activity

 Time: 10 minutes

→ • Click **Restart** from the summary menu.
• Choose the case by clicking on *Case 10: 25-year-old female—abdominal pain*.
• Listen to the dispatch, or read it in the right panel (or both).
• Click **Start**, and watch the entire video. Once the video has concluded, you are "on scene."
• Read the history log on the right side of the screen.

10. What barrier to communication was present on this case?

11. If the interpreter had not been present, could that have changed your clinical impression? Explain your answer.

12. What techniques could have been used to obtain information in the absence of an interpreter?

- Click **Quit Case**, and you will be taken to the summary menu.
- Click **Exit** to close the program, or **Restart** to continue with another lesson.

Documentation

Reading Assignment: Read Chapter 9, Documentation, in *EMT Prehospital Care,* Fourth Edition.

Case 1: 20-year-old male—difficulty breathing

Case 9: 22-year-old female—assault

Case 11: 32-year-old male—gunshot wounds

Case 13: 5-month-old male—unresponsive

Objectives:

On completion of this lesson, the student will be able to perform the following:

- Identify and document important information that should be included in your patient care report (PCR) from a scene size-up.

- Accurately and completely document subjective and objective findings, from dispatch through patient care, including primary assessment and interventions, as well as information from the rapid physical examination.

- Identify and apply reporting strategies you would use in special circumstances, such as calls when a crime may be involved.

EXERCISE 1

 CD-ROM Activity

 Time: 5 minutes

- Sign into the software by entering your name in the name tag and clicking **Enter**.
- Choose the case by clicking on *Case 1: 20-year-old male—difficulty breathing*.
- Listen to the dispatch, or read it in the right panel (or both).
- Click **Start**, and watch the entire video. Once the video has concluded, you are "on scene."
- Read the history log on the right side of the screen.
- You may use the **Look**, **Listen**, and **Feel** buttons, as well as determine pulse (P), blood pressure (BP), and respiration (R) readings before you answer the following questions.

1. Begin the narrative in the following table, providing the following information:

Aspect to Document	Answer
Chief complaint	
History	
Assessment	

- Click **Quit Case**, and you will be taken to the summary menu.

EXERCISE 2

 CD-ROM Activity

 Time: 15 minutes

2. Before you start the simulation, consider what you might observe at the scene of a crime involving a gunshot that would be considered important and should be included in the PCR. List three such observations:

- Click **Restart** from the summary menu.
- Choose the case by clicking on *Case 11: 32-year-old male—gunshot wounds*.
- Listen to the dispatch, or read it in the right panel (or both).
- Click **Start**, and begin watching the video.
- Click **Pause (❙❙)** as soon as the shirt is cut and opened.

3. Write the first few sentences that would appear in your PCR narrative for this patient.

4. Describe how you would document (in your PCR) the locations of the apparent bullet wounds that you observe after opening the shirt.

- Click **Play (▶)**. Once the video has concluded, you are "on scene."
- Read the history log on the right side of the screen.
- Perform the initial assessment and rapid physical examination using the **Assessment** buttons in the left panel.

5. Using the information gained, add these objective findings as you would document them in the narrative and vital signs areas of a PCR.

 • Click **Quit Case**, and you will be taken to the summary menu.

EXERCISE 3

 CD-ROM Activity

 Time: 15 minutes

• Click **Restart** from the summary menu.
• Choose the case by clicking on *Case 9: 22-year-old female—assault*.
• Listen to the dispatch, or read it in the right panel (or both).
• Click **Start**, and begin watching the video.
• Click **Pause (❚❚)** when the officer, Sergeant Campbell, completes her briefing.

6. Recognizing that this case will likely go to court and that your PCR will likely be evidence, consider what general observations about the patient environment might be considered important and should be included in the PCR. List two such observations:

a.

b.

• Click **Play (▶)** to resume the video.
• Click **Stop (■)** as soon as the patient finishes answering the question from the EMT.

7. List several observations you would include on your report that would describe the apparent psychological state of the patient, with the expectation that you would have to present this information in court.

8. You decide to perform a limited physical examination of the patient. How would your PCR indicate the fact that you did not conduct a physical examination of the patient specific to the sexual assault?

 • Click **Quit Case**, and you will be taken to the summary menu.

EXERCISE 4

 CD-ROM Activity

 Time: 10 minutes

 • Click **Restart** from the summary menu.
• Choose the case by clicking on *Case 13: 5-month-old male—unresponsive*.
• Listen to the dispatch, or read it in the right panel (or both).
• Click **Start**, and watch the entire video. Once the video has concluded, you are "on scene."
• Read the history log on the right side of the screen.
• Using the **Assessment** buttons in the left panel, perform the initial assessment, including *looking* and *feeling*, and begin treatment until cardiopulmonary resuscitation (CPR) is initiated.

9. Begin your report with the dispatch information, continuing through your application of cardio-pulmonary resuscitation (CPR) using basic life support equipment.

- Click **Quit Case**, and you will be taken to the summary menu.
→ - Click **Exit** to close the program, or **Restart** to continue with another lesson.

General Pharmacology

📖 **Reading Assignment:** Read Chapter 10, General Pharmacology, in *EMT Prehospital Care,* Fourth Edition.

Other Relevant Chapters:

- Chapter 12, Cardiovascular Emergencies
- Chapter 14, Allergies

Case 1: 20-year-old male—difficulty breathing

Case 14: 65-year-old male—difficulty breathing

Objectives:

On completion of this lesson, the student will be able to perform the following:

- Identify actions the emergency medical technician (EMT) should take before assisting with the administration of medications.
- Find key information for selected medications.
- Describe assessments the EMT should perform after administration of medications.

EXERCISE 1

 CD-ROM Activity

 Time: 15 minutes

- Sign into the software by entering your name in the name tag and clicking **Enter**.
- Choose the case by clicking on *Case 1: 20-year-old male—difficulty breathing*.
- Listen to the dispatch, or read it in the right panel (or both).
- Click **Start**, and watch the entire video. Once the video has concluded, you are "on scene."
- Read the history log on the right side of the screen.
- You may use the **Look**, **Listen**, and **Feel** buttons, as well as determine pulse, blood pressure, and respiration readings before you answer the following question.

Assume that the firefighters are EMTs.

1. Identify the information that the EMTs should have known about the drug they helped this patient to administer.

Drug Profile	Information Specific to Autoinjected Epinephrine
Indication	
Dose	
Administration	
Actions	
Contraindications	

2. How should the EMTs assess the patient after administering the drug?

3. What route did the EMTs use to administer the drug in this situation? Based on your answer, predict whether the drug will attain its full effect slowly or quickly.

 • Click **Quit Case**, and you will be taken to the summary menu.

EXERCISE 2

 CD-ROM Activity

 Time: 15 minutes

 • Click **Restart** from the summary menu.
- Choose the case by clicking on *Case 14: 65-year-old male—difficulty breathing*.
- Listen to the dispatch, or read it in the right panel (or both).
- Click **Start**, and begin watching the video.
- Read the history log on the right side of the screen.

After assessing this patient, you determine that you will assist him to administer his prescribed nitroglycerin tablets because of his chest pain.

4. What information should you know about this drug before you help the patient administer it?

Drug Profile	Information Specific to Nitroglycerin
Indication	

Drug Profile	Information Specific to Nitroglycerin
Dose	
Administration	
Actions	
Possible side effects	
Contraindications	

5. How should you assess the patient after giving him the drug?

6. What specific information should you check for on the label before you give this drug?

 • Click **Quit Case**, and you will be taken to the summary menu.
 • Click **Exit** to close the program, or **Restart** to continue with another lesson.

Respiratory Emergencies

Reading Assignment: Read Chapter 11, Respiratory Emergencies, in *EMT Prehospital Care,* Fourth Edition.

Other Relevant Chapters:
- Chapter 2, Well-Being of the EMT
- Chapter 6, Airway
- Chapter 7, Patient Assessment
- Chapter 8, Communications
- Chapter 9, Documentation
- Chapter 12, Cardiovascular Emergencies

Case 15: 42-year-old male—difficulty breathing

Objectives:

On completion of this lesson, the student will be able to perform the following:
- Form a clinical impression based on careful history and physical examination.
- Identify key interventions to treat this patient.
- Recognize appropriate safety interventions for emergency medical services (EMS) personnel in this case.

EXERCISE 1

 CD-ROM Activity

 Time: 30 minutes

- Sign into the software by entering your name in the name tag and clicking **Enter**.
- Choose the case by clicking on *Case 15: 42-year-old male—difficulty breathing*.
- Listen to the dispatch, or read it in the right panel (or both).
- Click **Start**, and watch the entire video. Once the video has concluded, you are "on scene."
- Read the history log on the right side of the screen.
- Perform your assessments and interventions using the buttons in the left panel. When you have determined that it is appropriate to begin transporting your patient to the hospital, click the **Load Patient** button. Continue your assessments and interventions en route to the hospital. When you have finished treating your patient, click the **Unload Patient** button. You will be taken to the summary menu.
- Click the **Log** button on the summary menu, and review your patient care as you answer the following questions.

1. List at least four possible causes of this patient's difficulty breathing, based on the initial information you have in the video of this call.

2. What are your highest priorities when caring for this patient?

3. Explain why you selected the oxygen device and flow rate that you did.

4. Was it appropriate for the EMTs to apply the masks? Explain your answer.

5. What other infection control measures should this crew take on this call?

6. The patient has tingling around his lips. Why do you think this is not hyperventilation related to an anxiety attack?

7. Complete a patient care report (PCR) for this call. (Use the following blank or one your instructor has given you.)

CHIEF COMPLAINT	
CURRENT MEDICATIONS	☐ NONE KNOWN
ALLERGIES (MEDICATIONS)	☐ NONE KNOWN
MEDICAL HISTORY	☐ MI ☐ CHF ☐ COPD ☐ ↑ BP ☐ DIABETES ☐ CANCER ☐ NONE KNOWN ☐ OTHER
NARRATIVE	

TIME	P	R	B/P	TREATMENT	RESPONSE/COMMENTS

• To save your log, click on the disk icon. To print your log, click on the printer icon.
 • Click **Menu** to return to the summary menu.
 • Click **Exit** to close the program, or **Restart** to continue with another lesson.

EXERCISE 2

 Summary Activity

Time: 10 minutes

8. How do you believe you handled this call?

9. Do you think you would change your actions if given the opportunity to complete the call again?

   If you said *yes*, what would you change and how do you think those changes would affect the patient?

 • Review your log with your instructor to see how it compares with the recommended care found in the implementation manual.

10. How did your care compare with what was recommended?

11. After reviewing the call, would you change anything on a subsequent call of this nature? Explain your answer.

Cardiovascular Emergencies

👓 **Reading Assignment:** Read Chapter 12, Cardiovascular Emergencies, in *EMT Prehospital Care,* Fourth Edition.

Other Relevant Chapters:

• Chapter 5, Lifting and Moving Patients

• Chapter 7, Patient Assessment

• Chapter 9, Documentation

Case 2: 56-year-old female—fell

Objectives:

On completion of this lesson, the student will be able to perform the following:

• Outline assessment techniques indicated to assess this patient appropriately.

• Transition care appropriately, based on changes in the patient's condition.

• Select appropriate interventions.

• Document care appropriately.

EXERCISE 1

 CD-ROM Activity

 Time: 30 minutes

- Sign into the software by entering your name in the name tag and clicking **Enter**.
- Choose the case by clicking on *Case 2: 56-year-old female—fell*.
- Listen to the dispatch, or read it in the right panel (or both).
- Click **Start**, and watch the entire video. Once the video has concluded, you are "on scene."
- Read the history log on the right side of the screen.

1. List your findings during the scene size-up. What actions would you take immediately, based on your findings during the scene size-up?

Elements of Size-Up	Findings	Actions Needed
Scene safety		
Mechanism of injury		
Nature of illness		
Number of patients		
Need for additional assistance		

2. What is your general impression of this patient based on the initial video encounter?

3. What illnesses or injuries do you need to rule out, based on your initial impression of the patient?

4. What challenge related to transportation is evident in the initial video images of this patient?

5. Describe strategies that you could use to manage the challenge(s) that you identified in the previous question.

 • Perform your assessments and interventions using the buttons in the left panel. When you have determined that it is appropriate to begin transporting your patient to the hospital, click the **Load Patient** button. Continue your assessments and interventions on the way to the hospital. When you have finished treating your patient, click the **Unload Patient** button. You will be taken to the summary menu.

• Click the **Log** button on the summary menu, and review your patient care as you answer the following questions.

6. Answer the following questions related to this patient's airway and breathing:

   a. State the initial oxygen device you used on this call and your reasons for using it.

   b. Describe your airway actions after the patient's condition changed (include positioning, noninvasive devices, ventilation, and oxygenation needed).

   c. If the patient is not breathing but has a pulse, describe the correct rate and depth of ventilations that you should deliver.

7. If you placed a Combitube in this patient, describe the significance of each of the assessment findings after placement and what action you would take after that assessment.

Assessment Finding	Significance	Actions Needed
When you ventilate through the pharyngeal lumen (#1), you observe the chest rise and fall, hear no sounds over the epigastrium, and auscultate breath sounds over both lungs.		
When you ventilate through the pharyngeal lumen (#1), you observe no chest rise and fall, and you hear bubbling over the epigastrium.		

Assessment Finding	Significance	Actions Needed
When you ventilate through the tracheal lumen (#2), you see the chest rise and fall, hear no bubbling over the epigastrium, and auscultate breath sounds over both lungs.		

8. You have delivered one shock with the automated external defibrillator (AED). Describe what the feedback means, and list your actions in each of the following situations:

   a. Two minutes after the shock is delivered, the machine reports, "No shock advised."

   b. Two minutes after the shock is delivered, the machine reports, "Shock advised, charging."

   c. One minute after the shock is delivered, the patient starts to move and you notice that she is breathing.

9. Would it be appropriate to terminate resuscitation in this case?

   If you answered *yes*, describe at what point in the resuscitation it would be appropriate. If you answered *no*, describe why this patient would not be an appropriate candidate for this decision.

10. Complete a patient care report (PCR) for this call. (Use the following blank or one your instructor has given you.)

CHIEF COMPLAINT	
CURRENT MEDICATIONS	☐ NONE KNOWN
ALLERGIES (MEDICATIONS)	☐ NONE KNOWN
MEDICAL HISTORY	☐ MI ☐ CHF ☐ COPD ☐ ↑ BP ☐ DIABETES ☐ CANCER ☐ NONE KNOWN ☐ OTHER
NARRATIVE	

TIME	P	R	B/P	TREATMENT	RESPONSE/COMMENTS

• To save your log, click on the disk icon. To print your log, click on the printer icon.
   • Click **Menu** to return to the summary menu.
   • Click **Exit** to close the program, or **Restart** to continue with another lesson.

EXERCISE 2

 Summary Activity

 Time: 10 minutes

11. How do you believe you handled this call?

12. Do you think you would change your actions if given the opportunity to complete the call again?

   If you said *yes*, what would you change and how do you think those changes would affect the patient?

  • Review your log with your instructor to see how it compares with the recommended care found in the implementation manual.

13. How did your care compare with what was recommended?

14. After reviewing the call, would you change anything on a subsequent call of this nature? Explain your answer.

Altered Mental Status

Reading Assignment: Read Chapter 13, Altered Mental Status, in *EMT Prehospital Care, Fourth Edition.*

Other Relevant Chapters:
- Chapter 7, Patient Assessment
- Chapter 9, Documentation
- Chapter 10, General Pharmacology

Case 4: 64-year-old male—unknown medical

Objectives:

On completion of this lesson, the student will be able to perform the following:
- Distinguish between key signs and symptoms to identify life threats in patients with altered level of consciousness.
- Identify appropriate interventions for the patient with altered level of consciousness.
- Perform assessment and reassessment in the appropriate sequence.
- Document the call appropriately.

.

EXERCISE 1

 CD-ROM Activity

 Time: 15 minutes

- Sign into the software by entering your name in the name tag and clicking **Enter**.
- Choose the case by clicking on *Case 4: 64-year-old male—unknown medical*.
- Listen to the dispatch, or read it in the right panel (or both).
- Click **Start**, and watch the entire video. Once the video has concluded, you are "on scene."
- Read the history log on the right side of the screen.
- Perform your assessments and interventions using the buttons in the left panel. When you have determined that it is appropriate to begin transporting your patient to the hospital, click the **Load Patient** button. Continue your assessments and interventions en route to the hospital. When you have finished treating your patient, click the **Unload Patient** button. You will be taken to the summary menu.
- Click the **Log** button on the summary menu, and review your patient care as you answer the following questions.

1. Based on the dispatch, initial scene observations, and family observations, state at least five possible causes of this patient's signs and symptoms. Describe why you chose each.

Possible Cause	Why You Suspect That Cause

2. If you elect to administer oral medication to this patient:

    a. Describe actions that you should take before giving it to ensure patient safety.

    b. How will you give it?

3. If the patient is unable to swallow and his level of consciousness is declining:

    a. What drug can you administer?

    b. By what route will you administer this drug?

    c. How does this drug increase blood glucose?

4. After you treat this patient, how will each of the following change if your patient is improving?

Sign or Symptom	Expected Change If Patient Improves
Pale, cold, clammy skin	
Confused	
Heart rate: 110 bpm (beats per minute)	

Sign or Symptom	Expected Change If Patient Improves
Slurred speech	

5. If you suspected that this patient were having a stroke, what additional signs or symptoms would you assess?

6. Describe some examples of effective communication that the emergency medical technicians demonstrated on this call.

7. Assume that this patient's daughter was interfering with your care by answering questions for the patient and standing between you and the patient, preventing you from examining him properly. What strategies could you and your partner use to solve that problem?

8. Complete a patient care report (PCR) for this call. (Use the following blank or one your instructor has given you.)

CHIEF COMPLAINT	
CURRENT MEDICATIONS	☐ NONE KNOWN
ALLERGIES (MEDICATIONS)	☐ NONE KNOWN
MEDICAL HISTORY	☐ MI ☐ CHF ☐ COPD ☐ ↑ BP ☐ DIABETES ☐ CANCER ☐ NONE KNOWN ☐ OTHER
NARRATIVE	

TIME	P	R	B/P	TREATMENT	RESPONSE/COMMENTS

• To save your log, click on the disk icon. To print your log, click on the printer icon.
• Click **Menu** to return to the summary menu.
• Click **Exit** to close the program, or **Restart** to continue with another lesson.

EXERCISE 2

 Summary Activity

Time: 10 minutes

9. How do you believe you handled this call?

10. Do you think you would change your actions if given the opportunity to complete the call again?

    If you said *yes*, what would you change and how do you think those changes would affect the patient?

• Review your log with your instructor to see how it compares with the recommended care found in the implementation manual.

11. How did your care compare with what was recommended?

12. After reviewing the call, would you change anything on a subsequent call of this nature?

Allergies

∞ **Reading Assignment:** Read Chapter 14, Allergies, in *EMT Prehospital Care,* Fourth Edition.

Other Relevant Chapters:
- Chapter 6, Airway
- Chapter 7, Patient Assessment
- Chapter 10, General Pharmacology

Case 1: 20-year-old male—difficulty breathing

Objectives:

On completion of this lesson, the student will be able to perform the following:
- Use an appropriate patient history and physical examination to find life threats.
- Deliver appropriate patient care in a sequence to maximize the patient's chance of recovery.
- Document the call accurately.

EXERCISE 1

 CD-ROM Activity

 Time: 40 minutes

 • Sign into the software by entering your name in the name tag and clicking **Enter**.
• Choose the case by clicking on *Case 1: 20-year-old male—difficulty breathing*.
• Listen to the dispatch, or read it in the right panel (or both).

1. What information would lead the dispatcher to state that the cause of the patient's difficulty breathing is related to an allergic reaction?

 • Click **Start**, and watch the entire video. Once the video has concluded, you are "on scene."
• Read the history log on the right side of the screen.

2. What do you observe on your initial scene size-up that may create some difficulty if the patient is transported?

3. Do the signs and symptoms that the emergency medical responders reported indicate that administration of the epinephrine auto-injector was appropriate? List the specific findings that justify your answer.

• Perform your assessments and interventions using the buttons in the left panel. When you have determined that it is appropriate to begin transporting your patient to the hospital, click the **Load Patient** button. Continue your assessments and interventions en route to the hospital. When you have finished treating your patient, click the **Unload Patient** button. You will be taken to the summary menu.
• Click the **Log** button on the summary menu, and review your patient care as you answer the following questions.

4. Explain why you selected the oxygen device and flow rate that you did.

5. What other assessment findings might you observe on this patient that indicate he is having an anaphylactic reaction?

6. Explain the effect that histamine has on the blood vessels during anaphylaxis.

7. What should you reassess often in the patient with anaphylaxis that could indicate the presence of a possible airway obstruction?

8. Explain why epinephrine, in the appropriate dose and route, will improve this patient's condition.

9. If the only medication you had available were the patient's albuterol, would it resolve *all* of the patient's signs and symptoms? Justify your response.

10. For each drug that was administered in this case, describe its desired action(s) and at least two side effects that you should expect.

Drug	Desired Action(s)	Side Effect(s)

11. On the following page, graph the systolic blood pressure (BP) and heart rate that you obtained in this call (consult your log). Then connect the data points so that each vital sign forms a line (see example). You can use blue ink for the systolic BP and red ink for the heart rate.

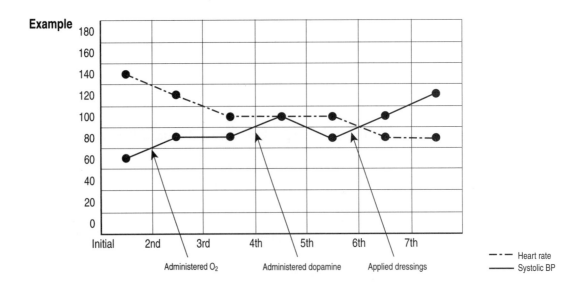

	Initial	2nd	3rd	4th	5th	6th	7th
180							
160							
140							
120							
100							
80							
60							
40							
20							
0							

12. Referring to the graph you just completed, answer the following questions:

   a. What trends do you observe?

   b. How did your interventions relate to the trends you observe?

   c. If the trend reversed at any point, how can you explain that variation?

13. Complete a patient care report (PCR) for this call. (Use the following blank or one your instructor has given you.)

CHIEF COMPLAINT	
CURRENT MEDICATIONS	☐ NONE KNOWN
ALLERGIES (MEDICATIONS)	☐ NONE KNOWN
MEDICAL HISTORY	☐ MI ☐ CHF ☐ COPD ☐ ↑ BP ☐ DIABETES ☐ CANCER ☐ NONE KNOWN ☐ OTHER
NARRATIVE	

TIME	P	R	B/P	TREATMENT	RESPONSE/COMMENTS

• To save your log, click on the disk icon. To print your log, click on the printer icon.
 • Click **Menu** to return to the summary menu.
 • Click **Exit** to close the program, or **Restart** to continue with another lesson.

EXERCISE 2

 Summary Activity

Time: 10 minutes

14. How do you believe you handled this call?

15. Do you think you would change your actions if given the opportunity to complete the call again?

    If you said *yes*, what would you change and how do you think those changes would affect the patient?

 • Review your log with your instructor to see how it compares with the recommended care found in the implementation manual.

16. How did your care compare with what was recommended?

17. After reviewing the call, would you change anything on a subsequent call of this nature? Explain your answer.

Poisoning and Overdoses

👓 **Reading Assignment:** Read Chapter 15, Poisoning and Overdoses, in *EMT Prehospital Care,* Fourth Edition.

Other Relevant Chapters:
- Chapter 5, Lifting and Moving Patients
- Chapter 6, Airway
- Chapter 7, Patient Assessment
- Chapter 9, Documentation
- Chapter 13, Altered Mental Status

Case 6: 16-year-old female—unknown medical

Objectives:

On completion of this lesson, the student will be able to perform the following:
- Identify priorities of care in an unresponsive patient based on a thorough patient assessment.
- Indicate appropriate patient management strategies.
- Evaluate the effectiveness of patient interventions.
- Identify resources to assist with patient care.

EXERCISE 1

 CD-ROM Activity

 Time: 30 minutes

- Sign into the software by entering your name in the name tag and clicking **Enter**.
- Choose the case by clicking on *Case 6: 16-year-old female—unknown medical.*
- Listen to the dispatch, or read it in the right panel (or both).
- Click **Start**, and watch the entire video. Once the video has concluded, you are "on scene."
- Read the history log on the right side of the screen.
- Perform your assessments and interventions using the buttons in the left panel. When you have determined that it is appropriate to begin transporting your patient to the hospital, click the **Load Patient** button. Continue your assessments and interventions on the way to the hospital. When you have finished treating your patient, click the **Unload Patient** button. You will be taken to the summary menu.
- Click the **Log** button on the summary menu, and review your patient care as you answer the following questions.

1. Explain your choice of airway/ventilation/oxygenation device.

2. What specific questions should you ask the family if you suspect the patient has taken an overdose?

3. List at least four possible causes of this patient's altered level of consciousness. What findings would you look for on your history or physical examination if you suspect that cause?

Cause	Findings to Look for in History or Physical Examination

4. Which of the following signs or symptoms of drug overdose did you observe in this patient? What intervention did you perform related to each sign or symptom that you identified?

Sign or Symptom	Yes/No	If Yes, Interventions Needed
Altered level of consciousness		

Sign or Symptom	Yes/No	If Yes, Interventions Needed
Seizures		
Agitation		
Fast heart rate		
Hypotension		
Hypertension		
Bradycardia		

5. Should you administer activated charcoal to this patient? Explain your answer.

6. If activated charcoal were indicated, outline the dose and the steps of administration of this drug.

7. What community resource can assist you to make treatment and transport decisions when caring for a patient with suspected poisoning?

8. Which of the following signs and symptoms of an opiate overdose did you observe in this patient?

Sign or Symptom	Observed in This Patient
Altered mental status	
Fresh or old needle marks (tracks)	
Pinpoint pupils	
Shallow, slow respirations	

9. What must you reevaluate during the ongoing assessment of this patient?

10. Graph the systolic blood pressure (BP) and heart rate that you obtained in this call (consult your log). Then connect the data points so that each vital sign forms a line (see example). You can use blue ink for the systolic BP and red ink for the heart rate.

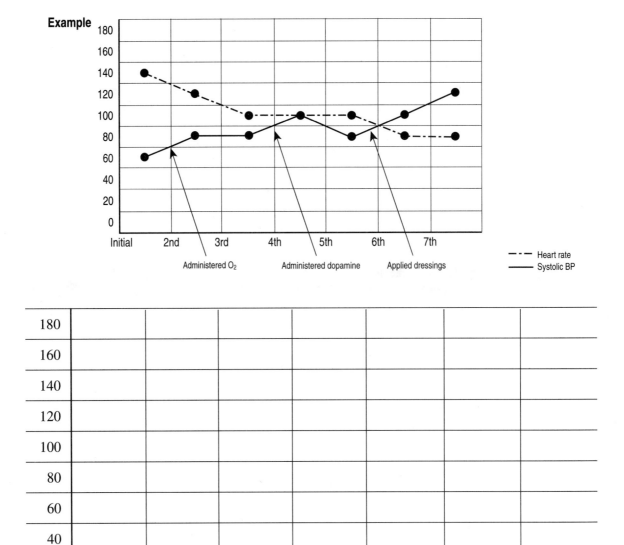

11. Referring to the graph you just completed, what trends do you observe?

12. Complete a patient care report (PCR) for this call. (Use the following blank or one your instructor has given you.)

CHIEF COMPLAINT	
CURRENT MEDICATIONS	☐ NONE KNOWN
ALLERGIES (MEDICATIONS)	☐ NONE KNOWN
MEDICAL HISTORY	☐ MI ☐ CHF ☐ COPD ☐ ↑ BP ☐ DIABETES ☐ CANCER ☐ NONE KNOWN ☐ OTHER
NARRATIVE	

TIME	P	R	B/P	TREATMENT	RESPONSE/COMMENTS

- To save your log, click on the disk icon. To print your log, click on the printer icon.
- Click **Menu** to return to the summary menu.
- Click **Exit** to close the program, or **Restart** to continue with another lesson.

EXERCISE 2

Summary Activity

Time: 10 minutes

13. How do you believe you handled this call?

14. Do you think you would change your actions if given the opportunity to complete the call again?

    If you said *yes*, what would you change and how do you think those changes would affect the patient?

- Review your log with your instructor to see how it compares with the recommended care found in the implementation manual.

15. How did your care compare with what was recommended?

16. After reviewing the call, would you change anything on a subsequent call of this nature? Explain your answer.

Environmental Emergencies I

———————————————————————————————

Reading Assignment: Read Chapter 16, Environmental Emergencies, in *EMT Prehospital Care,* Fourth Edition.

Other Relevant Chapters:

- Chapter 2, Well-Being of the EMT
- Chapter 6, Airway
- Chapter 7, Patient Assessment
- Chapter 9, Documentation
- Chapter 24, Injuries to the Head and Spine
- Chapter 25, Infants and Children

Case 7: 8-year-old male—submersion

Objectives:

On completion of this lesson, the student will be able to perform the following:

- Identify priorities of patient care, based on an appropriate patient assessment.
- Predict injuries, based on knowledge of mechanism of injury and relevant signs and symptoms.
- List appropriate measures for safe water rescue.

EXERCISE 1

  CD-ROM Activity

 Time: 15 minutes

→ • Sign into the software by entering your name in the name tag and clicking **Enter**.

• Choose the case by clicking on *Case 7: 8-year-old male—submersion*.

• Listen to the dispatch, or read it in the right panel (or both).

• Click **Start**, and watch the entire video. Once the video has concluded, you are "on scene."

• Read the history log on the right side of the screen.

• Perform your assessments and interventions using the buttons in the left panel. When you have determined that it is appropriate to begin transporting your patient to the hospital, click the **Load Patient** button. Continue your assessments and interventions on the way to the hospital. When you have finished treating your patient, click the **Unload Patient** button. You will be taken to the summary menu.

• Click the **Log** button on the summary menu, and review your patient care as you answer the following questions.

1. Was the care provided by the emergency medical responders (EMRs) appropriate? Explain your answer.

2. If you had suggestions to change the care provided by the EMRs, how would you address those concerns with them?

3. Explain why you selected the airway maneuvers, oxygen device, and flow rate that you did.

4. What factors will influence this patient's chance of survival?

5. Predict how the patient's condition might have changed if he had been rescued from the water 3 to 5 minutes later. Explain your answer.

6. Explain why the patient had the following signs or symptoms.

Sign or Symptom	Reason for Sign or Symptom
Rhonchi	
Unconsciousness	
Low oxygen saturation (SaO_2)	

7. What additional assessments and patient care measures would need to be taken if this event occurred on a day when the ambient temperature was 40° F (4° C)?

8. What actions would you take if the child were still submerged in the pool when you arrived?

   a. If the temperature were 86° F (30° C):

   b. If the temperature were 10° F (−12° C):

9. What risk factors for spinal cord injury does this patient have?

10. Are any of his vital sign findings consistent with spinal cord injury? Explain your answer.

11. Complete a patient care report (PCR) for this call. (Use the following blank or one your instructor has given you.)

CHIEF COMPLAINT	
CURRENT MEDICATIONS	☐ NONE KNOWN
ALLERGIES (MEDICATIONS)	☐ NONE KNOWN
MEDICAL HISTORY	☐ MI ☐ CHF ☐ COPD ☐ ↑ BP ☐ DIABETES ☐ CANCER ☐ NONE KNOWN ☐ OTHER
NARRATIVE	

TIME	P	R	B/P	TREATMENT	RESPONSE/COMMENTS

- To save your log, click on the disk icon. To print your log, click on the printer icon.
- Click **Menu** to return to the summary menu.
- Click **Exit** to close the program, or **Restart** to continue with another lesson.

EXERCISE 2

 Summary Activity

 Time: 10 minutes

12. How do you believe you handled this call?

13. Do you think you would change your actions if given the opportunity to complete the call again?

    If you said *yes*, what would you change and how do you think those changes would affect the patient?

- Review your log with your instructor to see how it compares with the recommended care found in the implementation manual.

14. How did your care compare with what was recommended?

15. After reviewing the call, would you change anything on a subsequent call of this nature? Explain your answer.

Environmental Emergencies II

✲ **Reading Assignment:** Read Chapter 16, Environmental Emergencies, in *EMT Prehospital Care,* Fourth Edition.

Other Relevant Chapters:

- Chapter 7, Patient Assessment
- Chapter 9, Documentation

Case 12: 57-year-old male—man down

Objectives:

On completion of this lesson, the student will be able to perform the following:

- Interpret information from the patient history and physical examination to identify life threats.
- Perform interventions in the correct sequence.
- Reassess the patient at the appropriate intervals.
- Document the call accurately.

EXERCISE 1

 CD-ROM Activity

 Time: 30 minutes

- Sign into the software by entering your name in the name tag and clicking **Enter**.
- Choose the case by clicking on *Case 12: 57-year-old male—man down*.
- Listen to the dispatch, or read it in the right panel (or both).
- Click **Start**, and watch the entire video. Once the video has concluded, you are "on scene."
- Read the history log on the right side of the screen.
- Perform your assessments and interventions using the buttons in the left panel. When you have determined that it is appropriate to begin transporting your patient to the hospital, click the **Load Patient** button. Continue your assessments and interventions en route to the hospital. When you have finished treating your patient, click the **Unload Patient** button. You will be taken to the summary menu.
- Click the **Log** button on the summary menu and review your patient care as you answer the following questions.

1. Describe what you discovered in your scene size-up, and list any additional actions to be taken immediately, based on the information you found.

2. Explain why you selected the oxygen device and flow rate that you did.

3. What noninvasive interventions should you perform before transport? Explain the rationale for performing them.

4. What type of patient is at high risk for this condition? Does this patient have any of those risk factors?

5. Explain the significance of each of the following findings from your patient assessment.

Sign or Symptom	Significance
Diaphoresis	
Respiratory rate: 32 breaths/min	
Heart rate: 146 bpm (beats per minute)	

6. If you do not treat your patient quickly, how might his illness progress?

7. How does shivering increase body temperature?

8. What environmental factors contribute to this type of illness?

9. If an advanced life support (ALS) unit is available, why should you call them?

10. Complete a patient care report (PCR) for this call. (Use the following blank or one your instructor has given you.)

CHIEF COMPLAINT	
CURRENT MEDICATIONS	☐ NONE KNOWN
ALLERGIES (MEDICATIONS)	☐ NONE KNOWN
MEDICAL HISTORY	☐ MI ☐ CHF ☐ COPD ☐ ↑ BP ☐ DIABETES ☐ CANCER ☐ NONE KNOWN ☐ OTHER
NARRATIVE	

TIME	P	R	B/P	TREATMENT	RESPONSE/COMMENTS

• To save your log, click on the disk icon. To print your log, click on the printer icon.
• Click **Menu** to return to the summary menu.
• Click **Exit** to close the program, or **Restart** to continue with another lesson.

EXERCISE 2

 Summary Activity

Time: 10 minutes

11. How do you believe you handled this call?

12. Do you think you would change your actions if given the opportunity to complete the call again?

   If you said *yes*, what would you change and how do you think those changes would affect the patient?

 • Review your log with your instructor to see how it compares with the recommended care found in the implementation manual.

13. How did your care compare with what was recommended?

14. After reviewing the call, would you change anything on a subsequent call of this nature? Explain your answer.

Behavioral Emergencies

👓 **Reading Assignment:** Read Chapter 17, Behavioral Emergencies, in *EMT Prehospital Care*, Fourth Edition.

Other Relevant Chapters:

- Chapter 2, Well-Being of the EMT
- Chapter 7, Patient Assessment
- Chapter 9, Documentation
- Chapter 13, Altered Mental Status

Case 8: 38-year-old male—suicide attempt

Objectives:

On completion of this lesson, the student will be able to perform the following:

- Demonstrate knowledge of appropriate techniques to restrain a patient physically.
- Describe appropriate measures to monitor a restrained patient.
- Outline techniques to distinguish medical versus psychiatric causes of behavioral illness.
- State appropriate techniques to communicate with a patient with a behavioral emergency.

EXERCISE 1

 CD-ROM Activity

 Time: 30 minutes

- Sign into the software by entering your name in the name tag and clicking **Enter**.
- Choose the case by clicking on *Case 8: 38-year-old male—suicide attempt*.
- Listen to the dispatch, or read it in the right panel (or both).
- Click **Start**, and watch the entire video. Once the video has concluded, you are "on scene."
- Read the history log on the right side of the screen.
- Perform your assessments and interventions using the buttons in the left panel. When you have determined that it is appropriate to begin transporting your patient to the hospital, click the **Load Patient** button. Continue your assessments and interventions en route to the hospital. When you have finished treating your patient, click the **Unload Patient** button. You will be taken to the summary menu.
- Click the **Log** button on the summary menu, and review your patient care as you answer the following questions.

1. Why should you stage (and not approach) the scene on this type of dispatch until the police signal that the scene is safe?

2. How did the police place the patient on the stretcher? Is it acceptable for you to leave the patient restrained in that manner? Explain your answer.

3. Describe how you would position the patient for transport.

4. Were the police officer's initial comments to the patient appropriate? Explain your answer.

5. What type of abnormal communication did you observe this patient make?

6. What other signs or symptoms did you observe that could indicate that this patient is violent?

7. During your assessment of this patient, you will need to rule out any medical causes of his bizarre behavior. List at least four possible medical causes of altered mental status, as well as one or two specific signs or symptoms that you will assess to rule them out.

Organic Cause	Signs or Symptoms to Assess

Organic Cause	Signs or Symptoms to Assess

8. What nonpharmacologic measures can you take to calm this patient's behavior during your care and transportation?

9. What must you do before physically restraining a patient?

10. What specific patient assessment is necessary for a patient who is restrained?

11. Complete a patient care report (PCR) for this call. (Use the following blank or one your instructor has given you.)

CHIEF COMPLAINT	
CURRENT MEDICATIONS	☐ NONE KNOWN
ALLERGIES (MEDICATIONS)	☐ NONE KNOWN
MEDICAL HISTORY	☐ MI ☐ CHF ☐ COPD ☐ ↑ BP ☐ DIABETES ☐ CANCER ☐ NONE KNOWN ☐ OTHER
NARRATIVE	

TIME	P	R	B/P	TREATMENT	RESPONSE/COMMENTS

• To save your log, click on the disk icon. To print your log, click on the printer icon.
- Click **Menu** to return to the summary menu.
- Click **Exit** to close the program, or **Restart** to continue with another lesson.

EXERCISE 2

 Summary Activity

 Time: 10 minutes

12. How do you believe you handled this call?

13. Do you think you would change your actions if given the opportunity to complete the call again?

   If you said *yes*, what would you change and how do you think those changes would affect the patient?

 • Review your log with your instructor to see how it compares with the recommended care found in the implementation manual.

14. How did your care compare with what was recommended?

15. After reviewing the call, would you change anything on a subsequent call of this nature? Explain your answer.

Abuse and Assault

Reading Assignment: Read Chapter 18, Abuse and Assault, in *EMT Prehospital Care,* Fourth Edition.

Case 3: 7-year-old female—seizure

Case 9: 22-year-old female—assault

Case 10: 25-year-old female—abdominal pain

Case 14: 65-year-old male—difficulty breathing

Objectives:

On completion of this lesson, the student will be able to perform the following:

- Distinguish between types of abuse.
- Outline risk factors for abuse and neglect.
- Apply assessment principles to detect injuries associated with abuse.
- Describe appropriate communication strategies when caring for patients who have been abused or assaulted.
- Discuss legal obligations of the emergency medical technician (EMT) when caring for patients who have been abused or neglected.

EXERCISE 1

 CD-ROM Activity

 Time: 20 minutes

 • Sign into the software by entering your name in the name tag and clicking **Enter**.
 • Choose the case by clicking on *Case 3: 7-year-old female—seizure*.
 • Listen to the dispatch, or read it in the right panel (or both).
 • Click **Start**, and watch the entire video. Once the video has concluded, you are "on scene."
 • Read the history log on the right side of the screen.

1. What features of this call increase your suspicion that abuse or neglect may be present in this home?

2. Using the initial history and scene size-up provided in the scenario, explain why the features listed below would or would not increase your suspicion of abuse in this child.

Initial History and Scene Size-Up	Indicates Risk of Abuse? (Yes/No/Uncertain)	Explain Your Rationale

• Click **Quit Case**, and you will be taken to the summary menu.

EXERCISE 2

 CD-ROM Activity

 Time: 15 minutes

 • Click **Restart** from the summary menu.
• Choose the case by clicking on *Case 10: 25-year-old female—abdominal pain*.
• Listen to the dispatch, or read it in the right panel (or both).
• Click **Start**, and watch the entire video. Once the video has concluded, you are "on scene."
• Read the history log on the right side of the screen.

3. What increases this patient's risk for domestic violence?

4. What type of trauma would you assess for if you suspect violence is a cause of this patient's headache and abdominal pain?

5. How should you question her if you find injuries that suggest abuse?

6. What should you tell her if she says her husband kicked her in the head and stomach but she does not wish to be transported because she says her husband "was crying and said he was sorry and promised it will never happen again?"

 • Click **Quit Case**, and you will be taken to the summary menu.

EXERCISE 3

 CD-ROM Activity

 Time: 15 minutes

- Click **Restart** from the summary menu.
- Choose the case by clicking on *Case 9: 22-year-old female—assault*.
- Listen to the dispatch, or read it in the right panel (or both).
- Click **Start**, and watch the entire video. Once the video has concluded, you are "on scene."
- Read the history log on the right side of the screen.

7. Assume that this patient's only complaint is that she was sexually assaulted. She asks if she can take a shower before you transport her for evaluation at the hospital. What should you say?

8. What communication techniques should you use or avoid so the person who has been sexually assaulted does not feel that you are blaming her for the assault?

- Click **Quit Case**, and you will be taken to the summary menu.

EXERCISE 4

 CD-ROM Activity

 Time: 15 minutes

- Click **Restart** from the summary menu.
- Choose the case by clicking on *Case 14: 65-year-old male—difficulty breathing*.
- Listen to the dispatch, or read it in the right panel (or both).
- Click **Start**, and watch the entire video. Once the video has concluded, you are "on scene."
- Read the history log on the right side of the screen.

9. Do you observe any signs of neglect in the initial video of this case? If you answered *yes*, explain what you found. If you answered *no*, explain why.

10. You are concerned because the patient appears very thin. How will you try to determine whether he has adequate nutrition?

11. The neighbors express concern that the patient's adult son seems to be taking advantage of his father. He has been having his father purchase expensive things for him, and the patient has confided that he is running out of money for food. If these allegations are true, what type of abuse is this? What should you do about it?

➡ • Click **Quit Case**, and you will be taken to the summary menu.
  • Click **Exit** to close the program, or **Restart** to continue with another lesson.

Obstetrics and Gynecology

Reading Assignment: Read Chapter 19, Obstetrics and Gynecology, in *EMT Prehospital Care, Fourth Edition.*

Other Relevant Chapters:

- Chapter 7, Patient Assessment
- Chapter 8, Communications
- Chapter 9, Documentation
- Chapter 13, Altered Mental Status

Case 10: 25-year-old female—abdominal pain

Objectives:

On completion of this lesson, the student will be able to perform the following:

- Recognize and treat complications of pregnancy.
- Anticipate signs and symptoms that may develop in a patient with complications of pregnancy.
- Describe management of seizures in a pregnant patient.

EXERCISE 1

 CD-ROM Activity

 Time: 30 minutes

- Sign into the software by entering your name in the name tag and clicking **Enter**.
- Choose the case by clicking on *Case 10: 25-year-old female—abdominal pain*.
- Listen to the dispatch, or read it in the right panel (or both).
- Click **Start**, and watch the entire video. Once the video has concluded, you are "on scene."
- Read the history log on the right side of the screen.
- Perform your assessments and interventions using the buttons in the left panel. When you have determined that it is appropriate to begin transporting your patient to the hospital, click the **Load Patient** button. Continue your assessments and interventions en route to the hospital. When you have finished treating your patient, click the **Unload Patient** button. You will be taken to the summary menu.
- Click the **Log** button on the summary menu, and review your patient care as you answer the following questions.

1. What communication barrier did you face on this call?

2. How would you have handled this barrier if the patient's friend were not present on the call?

3. Explain why you selected the oxygen device and flow rate that you did.

4. This patient says she has "1 month to go" in her pregnancy. If this is accurate, how many weeks into her pregnancy is she?

5. Explain how the following body functions are affected by normal pregnancy, as well as whether this patient's vital signs are what should be expected at this stage of pregnancy.

Body Function	Expected Change in Pregnancy	This Patient
Cardiovascular function		
Respiratory function		
Blood pressure (BP)		

6. What condition do you believe this patient has?

7. What additional physical findings might you observe in this patient that confirm your initial clinical impression?

8. Important considerations for transport of this patient exist.

   a. What is an acceptable position for transport of this patient?

   b. Discuss measures that should be taken during transport for supportive care of this patient.

   c. Describe how you will determine the appropriate transport destination for this patient.

9. What care should you provide if this patient has a seizure on the way to the hospital?

10. This patient has severe abdominal pain not associated with labor.

   a. What is a possible life-threatening complication of pregnancy that can cause this pain?

b. What signs and symptoms related to her pain will you look for?

c. What are the implications of this pain to the mother and fetus?

11. If the blood pressure continues to increase, what other life-threatening complications may occur?

12. If the patient were suddenly to develop labor and deliver the newborn in the field, what initial measures would you take to resuscitate the newborn?

a. If the infant appeared normal:

b. If the infant were taking slow, gasping respirations:

c. If the infant's heart rate were 60 beats per minute (bpm):

13. Complete a patient care report (PCR) for this call. (Use the following blank or one your instructor has given you.)

CHIEF COMPLAINT	
CURRENT MEDICATIONS	☐ NONE KNOWN
ALLERGIES (MEDICATIONS)	☐ NONE KNOWN
MEDICAL HISTORY	☐ MI ☐ CHF ☐ COPD ☐ ↑ BP ☐ DIABETES ☐ CANCER ☐ NONE KNOWN ☐ OTHER
NARRATIVE	

TIME	P	R	B/P	TREATMENT	RESPONSE/COMMENTS

• To save your log, click on the disk icon. To print your log, click on the printer icon.
  • Click **Menu** to return to the summary menu.
  • Click **Exit** to close the program, or **Restart** to continue with another lesson.

EXERCISE 2

  Summary Activity

  Time: 10 minutes

14. How do you believe you handled this call?

15. Do you think you would change your actions if given the opportunity to complete the call again?

    If you said *yes*, what would you change, and how do you think your changes would affect the patient?

  • Review your log with your instructor to see how it compares with the recommended care found in the implementation manual.

16. How did your care compare with what was recommended?

17. After reviewing the call, would you change anything on a subsequent call of this nature? Explain your answer.

Bleeding and Shock

📖 **Reading Assignment:** Read Chapter 20, Bleeding and Shock, in *EMT Prehospital Care,* Fourth Edition.

Other Relevant Chapters:
- Chapter 2, Well-Being of the EMT
- Chapter 6, Airway
- Chapter 7, Patient Assessment
- Chapter 9, Documentation

Case 5: 40-year-old male—vomiting blood

Objectives:

On completion of this lesson, the student will be able to perform the following:

- Perform an appropriate patient history and physical examination to establish clinical priorities of care.
- Deliver appropriate patient care in a proper sequence to maximize the patient's chance for recovery.
- Identify appropriate interventions for a patient who is vomiting blood.
- Anticipate appropriate personal protective equipment (PPE) that would be needed on a call with a patient who is vomiting blood.

EXERCISE 1

 CD-ROM Activity

 Time: 30 minutes to complete

- Sign into the software by entering your name in the name tag and clicking **Enter**.
- Choose the case by clicking on *Case 5: 40-year-old male—vomiting blood*.
- Listen to the dispatch, or read it in the right panel (or both).
- Click **Start**, and watch the entire video. Once the video has concluded, you are "on scene."
- Read the history log on the right side of the screen.
- Perform your assessments and interventions using the buttons in the left panel. When you have determined that it is appropriate to begin transporting your patient to the hospital, click the **Load Patient** button. Continue your assessments and interventions en route to the hospital. When you have finished treating your patient, click the **Unload Patient** button. You will be taken to the summary menu.
- Click the **Log** button on the summary menu, and review your patient care as you answer the following questions.

1. What are your priorities in the care of this patient?

2. Complete the following information related to the steps in your primary assessment of this patient.

Action	Finding	Action Needed (If Any)
Develop a general impression		
Determine if life threats exist		

Action	Finding	Action Needed (If Any)
Assess level of consciousness		
Assess airway		
Assess breathing		
Assess circulation		
Assess for major bleeding		

Action	Finding	Action Needed (If Any)
Manage bleeding		
Assess perfusion		

3. Explain why you selected the oxygen device and flow rate that you did.

4. What safety measures should you and your partner take, based on your initial impression of the patient?

5. What airway equipment should you have ready after you perform your initial assessment?

6. In what position would you place this patient for transport? Explain your answer.

7. List four signs or symptoms of shock that you identified when assessing this patient. Explain the cause of each sign or symptom.

Sign or Symptom	Cause

8. List the components of your reassessment of the patient.

9. How often should you reassess this patient?

10. What should you include in your documentation related to this patient's bleeding?

11. If he describes his pain as severe epigastric pain, what organs would you suspect are involved?

12. What specific signs or symptoms lead you to believe that this is a gastrointestinal problem?

13. Complete a patient care report (PCR) for this call. (Use the following blank or one your instructor has given you.)

CHIEF COMPLAINT	
CURRENT MEDICATIONS	☐ NONE KNOWN
ALLERGIES (MEDICATIONS)	☐ NONE KNOWN
MEDICAL HISTORY	☐ MI ☐ CHF ☐ COPD ☐ ↑ BP ☐ DIABETES ☐ CANCER ☐ NONE KNOWN ☐ OTHER
NARRATIVE	

TIME	P	R	B/P	TREATMENT	RESPONSE/COMMENTS

- To save your log, click on the disk icon. To print your log, click on the printer icon.
- Click **Menu** to return to the summary menu.
- Click **Exit** to close the program, or **Restart** to continue with another lesson.

EXERCISE 2

Summary Activity

Time: 10 minutes

14. How do you believe you handled this call?

15. Do you think you would change your actions if given the opportunity to complete the call again?

    If you said *yes*, what would you change and how do you think those changes would affect the patient?

- Review your log with your instructor to see how it compares with the recommended care found in the implementation manual.

16. How did your care compare with what was recommended?

17. After reviewing the call, would you change anything on a subsequent call of this nature?

 • Click **Quit Case**, and you will be taken to the summary menu.
• Click **Exit** to close the program, or **Restart** to continue with another lesson.

Multisystem Trauma

Reading Assignment: Read Chapter 20, Bleeding and Shock; Chapter 21, Soft Tissue Injuries; Chapter 22, Chest and Abdominal Emergencies; and Chapter 24, Injuries to the Head and Spine, in *EMT Prehospital Care,* Fourth Edition.

Other Relevant Chapters:
- Chapter 2, Well-Being of the EMT
- Chapter 3, Medicolegal and Ethical Issues
- Chapter 6, Airway
- Chapter 7, Patient Assessment
- Chapter 9, Documentation

Case 11: 32-year-old male—gunshot wounds

Objectives:
On completion of this lesson, the student will be able to perform the following:
- Demonstrate appropriate actions to take when responding to a patient who has been shot.
- Predict the injuries from penetrating trauma, based on knowledge of anatomy and physiology.
- Manage life threats, including airway, breathing, and circulatory problems for the patient with penetrating trauma.

EXERCISE 1

 CD-ROM Activity

 Time: 30 minutes

- Sign into the software by entering your name in the name tag and clicking **Enter**.
- Choose the case by clicking on *Case 11: 32-year-old male—gunshot wounds*.
- Listen to the dispatch, or read it in the right panel (or both).
- Click **Start**, and watch the entire video. Once the video has concluded, you are "on scene."
- Read the history log on the right side of the screen.
- Perform your assessments and interventions using the buttons in the left panel. When you have determined that it is appropriate to begin transporting your patient to the hospital, click the **Load Patient** button. Continue your assessments and interventions en route to the hospital. When you have finished treating your patient, click the **Unload Patient** button. You will be taken to the summary menu.
- Click the **Log** button on the summary menu, and review your patient care as you answer the following questions.

1. How do you know that the scene is safe and you may approach the patient?

2. What immediate life threats did you identify in this patient?

3. What type of dressing would you apply to each wound? Discuss your rationale for the application of each.

Wound	Dressing	Rationale
Neck		

Wound	Dressing	Rationale
Chest		
Abdomen		

4. What causes of shock did you identify in this patient?

5. What signs, symptoms, or physical findings helped you form a clinical impression of the type of shock the patient is experiencing?

6. Explain the rationale for the airway, ventilation, and oxygenation choices you made for this patient.

7. Based on the location of the gunshot wounds, as well as the patient's signs and symptoms, predict which organs or significant body structures each bullet injured.

   a. Neck:

   b. Chest:

   c. Abdomen:

8. List at least three measures you should take to preserve evidence on this call.

9. Complete a patient care report (PCR) for this call. (Use the following blank or one your instructor has given you.)

CHIEF COMPLAINT	
CURRENT MEDICATIONS	☐ NONE KNOWN
ALLERGIES (MEDICATIONS)	☐ NONE KNOWN
MEDICAL HISTORY	☐ MI ☐ CHF ☐ COPD ☐ ↑ BP ☐ DIABETES ☐ CANCER ☐ NONE KNOWN ☐ OTHER
NARRATIVE	

TIME	P	R	B/P	TREATMENT	RESPONSE/COMMENTS

• To save your log, click on the disk icon. To print your log, click on the printer icon.
- Click **Menu** to return to the summary menu.
- Click **Exit** to close the program, or **Restart** to continue with another lesson.

EXERCISE 2

 Summary Activity

 Time: 10 minutes

10. How do you believe you handled this call?

11. Do you think you would change your actions if given the opportunity to complete the call again?

    If you said *yes*, what would you change and how do you think those changes would affect the patient?

 • Review your log with your instructor to see how it compares with the recommended care found in the implementation manual.

12. How did your care compare with what was recommended?

13. After reviewing the call, would you change anything on a subsequent call of this nature? Explain your answer.

Soft Tissue Injuries

📖 **Reading Assignment:** Read Chapter 21, Soft Tissue Injuries, in *EMT Prehospital Care,* Fourth Edition.

Other Relevant Chapters:
- Chapter 2, Well-Being of the EMT
- Chapter 3, Medicolegal and Ethical Issues
- Chapter 7, Patient Assessment
- Chapter 8, Communications
- Chapter 9, Documentation
- Chapter 18, Abuse and Assault
- Chapter 19, Obstetrics and Gynecology
- Chapter 24, Injuries to the Head and Spine

Case 9: 22-year-old female—assault

Objectives:

On completion of this lesson, the student will be able to perform the following:
- Outline care for the physical and psychological needs of a patient who has been subjected to physical, sexual, or emotional abuse.
- Assess burns to determine the depth, size, and severity of the thermal injury.
- Outline the appropriate care of a burn injury.
- Discuss how to integrate crime scene preservation into the care of the rape victim.
- Document the call appropriately.

EXERCISE 1

 CD-ROM Activity

 Time: 30 minutes

- Sign into the software by entering your name in the name tag and clicking **Enter**.
- Choose the case by clicking on *Case 9: 22-year-old female—assault*.
- Listen to the dispatch, or read it in the right panel (or both).
- Click **Start**, and watch the entire video. Once the video has concluded, you are "on scene."
- Read the history log on the right side of the screen.
- Perform your assessments and interventions using the buttons in the left panel. When you have determined that it is appropriate to begin transporting your patient to the hospital, click the **Load Patient** button. Continue your assessments and interventions en route to the hospital. When you have finished treating your patient, click the **Unload Patient** button. You will be taken to the summary menu.
- Click the **Log** button on the summary menu, and review your patient care as you answer the following questions.

1. Based on the initial information you received from dispatch and your primary assessment, list at least four injuries or illnesses that you may encounter on this call.

2. As you enter the room to assess and manage the patient, what are your priorities?

3. Describe why you believe the patient should or should not have spinal immobilization.

4. Describe the detailed assessment you would perform on this patient's jaw.

5. Explain your rationale for the genital examination you should perform on this patient.

6. What are your goals related to the patient's complaint of sexual assault?

7. Describe signs or symptoms that would lead you to suspect that this patient has an inhalation injury.

8. Calculate the extent (percent of body surface area [BSA]) of the burn injury.

9. What is the depth of the burn injury? Explain your answer.

10. Will this patient require care at a burn center? Explain your answer.

11. How will you cover the burn injury in this patient to help relieve her pain?

12. Complete a patient care report (PCR) for this call. (Use the following blank or one your instructor has given you.)

CHIEF COMPLAINT	
CURRENT MEDICATIONS	☐ NONE KNOWN
ALLERGIES (MEDICATIONS)	☐ NONE KNOWN
MEDICAL HISTORY	☐ MI ☐ CHF ☐ COPD ☐ ↑ BP ☐ DIABETES ☐ CANCER ☐ NONE KNOWN ☐ OTHER
NARRATIVE	

TIME	P	R	B/P	TREATMENT	RESPONSE/COMMENTS

• To save your log, click on the disk icon. To print your log, click on the printer icon.
 • Click **Menu** to return to the summary menu.
 • Click **Exit** to close the program, or **Restart** to continue with another lesson.

EXERCISE 2

 Summary Activity

Time: 10 minutes

13. How do you believe you handled this call?

14. Do you think you would change your actions if given the opportunity to complete the call again?

    If you said *yes*, what would you change and how do you think those changes would affect the patient?

 • Review your log with your instructor to see how it compares with the recommended care found in the implementation manual.

15. How did your care compare with what was recommended?

16. After reviewing the call, would you change anything on a subsequent call of this nature? Explain your answer.

Infants and Children I

✍ **Reading Assignment:** Read Chapter 25, Infants and Children, in *EMT Prehospital Care,* Fourth
Edition.

Other Relevant Chapters:
- Chapter 2, Well-Being of the EMT
- Chapter 3, Medicolegal and Ethical Issues
- Chapter 6, Airway
- Chapter 7 Patient Assessment
- Chapter 8, Communications
- Chapter 9, Documentation
- Chapter 12, Cardiovascular Emergencies

Case 13: 5-month-old male—unresponsive

Objectives:
On completion of this lesson, the student will be able to perform the following:
- Perform a rapid assessment to determine priorities of care in a critically ill child.
- Deliver effective care in a critically ill child.
- Use effective communication techniques to obtain an accurate history and to facilitate a therapeutic
relationship with a critically ill child's parents.

EXERCISE 1

 CD-ROM Activity

 Time: 30 minutes

- Sign into the software by entering your name in the name tag and clicking **Enter**.
- Choose the case by clicking on *Case 13: 5-month-old male—unresponsive*.
- Listen to the dispatch, or read it in the right panel (or both).
- Click **Start**, and watch the entire video. Once the video has concluded, you are "on scene."
- Read the history log on the right side of the screen.
- Perform your assessments and interventions using the buttons in the left panel. When you have determined that it is appropriate to begin transporting your patient to the hospital, click the **Load Patient** button. Continue your assessments and interventions en route to the hospital. When you have finished treating your patient, click the **Unload Patient** button. You will be taken to the summary menu.
- Click the **Log** button on the summary menu, and review your patient care as you answer the following questions.

1. Name at least four situations that you thought might be present on this call after you heard the dispatch information.

2. What physical findings on arrival would indicate that you should NOT attempt to resuscitate a pulseless, nonbreathing newborn, infant, or child?

3. Describe your technique for chest compressions on this infant, including rate, depth, and hand position.

4. Should you use the automated external defibrillator (AED) on this patient? Explain your answer.

5. Describe considerations in positioning the airway of this patient.

6. Explain why you selected the oxygen device and flow rate that you did.

7. What additional physical findings are you looking for when you perform your focused history and physical examination?

8. Describe some general communication techniques you can use if the patient's mother approaches you at the hospital and asks about the infant's condition.

9. What will you say if she asks, "How's my baby?"

10. Complete a patient care report (PCR) for this call. (Use the following blank or one your instructor has given you.)

CHIEF COMPLAINT	
CURRENT MEDICATIONS	☐ NONE KNOWN
ALLERGIES (MEDICATIONS)	☐ NONE KNOWN
MEDICAL HISTORY	☐ MI ☐ CHF ☐ COPD ☐ ↑ BP ☐ DIABETES ☐ CANCER ☐ NONE KNOWN ☐ OTHER
NARRATIVE	

TIME	P	R	B/P	TREATMENT	RESPONSE/COMMENTS

• To save your log, click on the disk icon. To print your log, click on the printer icon.
- Click **Menu** to return to the summary menu.
- Click **Exit** to close the program, or **Restart** to continue with another lesson.

EXERCISE 2

 Summary Activity

Time: 10 minutes

11. How do you believe you handled this call?

12. Do you think you would change your actions if given the opportunity to complete the call again?

   If you said *yes*, what would you change and how do you think those changes would affect the patient?

 • Review your log with your instructor to see how it compares with the recommended care found in the implementation manual.

13. How did your care compare with what was recommended?

14. After reviewing the call, would you change anything on a subsequent call of this nature? Explain your answer.

Infants and Children II

👓 **Reading Assignment:** Read Chapter 25, Infants and Children, in *EMT Prehospital Care,* Fourth Edition.

Other Relevant Chapters:
- Chapter 2, Well-Being of the EMT
- Chapter 6, Airway
- Chapter 7, Patient Assessment
- Chapter 9, Documentation
- Chapter 13, Altered Mental Status

Case 3: 7-year-old female—seizure

Objectives:
On completion of this lesson, the student will be able to perform the following:
- Describe the reasons for specific scene safety considerations on this call.
- Perform appropriate patient assessments in the correct sequence.
- Interpret signs and symptoms to identify life-threatening conditions.
- Identify appropriate interventions.
- Evaluate the effectiveness of patient interventions.

EXERCISE 1

 CD-ROM Activity

  Time: 30 minutes

- Sign into the software by entering your name in the name tag and clicking **Enter**.
- Choose the case by clicking on *Case 3: 7-year-old female—seizure*.
- Listen to the dispatch, or read it in the right panel (or both).

1. What illness or injuries come to mind, based on the dispatch information only?

2. Would the age of the patient influence your previous answer?

- Click **Start**, and watch the entire video. Once the video has concluded, you are "on scene."
- Read the history log on the right side of the screen.
- Perform your assessments and interventions using the buttons in the left panel. When you have determined that it is appropriate to begin transporting your patient to the hospital, click the **Load Patient** button. Continue your assessments and interventions en route to the hospital. When you have finished treating your patient, click the **Unload Patient** button. You will be taken to the summary menu.
- Click the **Log** button on the summary menu, and review your patient care as you answer the following questions.

3. Explain why you performed the airway interventions you selected.

4. Explain the rationale for the safety measures the crew took on this call.

5. What are some possible explanations for the behavior of the child's father?

6. State whether her initial vital sign findings are normal or abnormal. If you say *abnormal*, list what you would expect for normal.

Finding	Normal or Abnormal	Normal Findings
Blood pressure (BP): 60/36 mm Hg		
Pulse (P): 200 bpm (beats per minute)		
Respiratory rate: not measurable		
Saturation of peripheral oxygen (SpO$_2$): 88%		

7. List at least three illnesses or injuries that could cause this child's presenting signs and symptoms. Explain why you chose these.

Injury or Illness	Factors Present That Indicated This Problem

8. If the patient's mother says her daughter is diabetic and you suspect hypoglycemia, should you give her oral glucose paste or gel? Explain your answer.

9. Based on your knowledge related to the child's illness, what should you do if the patient's mother asks you, "Is my daughter going to be okay?"

10. Complete a patient care report (PCR) for this call. (Use the following blank or one your instructor has given you.)

CHIEF COMPLAINT	
CURRENT MEDICATIONS	☐ NONE KNOWN
ALLERGIES (MEDICATIONS)	☐ NONE KNOWN
MEDICAL HISTORY	☐ MI ☐ CHF ☐ COPD ☐ ↑ BP ☐ DIABETES ☐ CANCER ☐ NONE KNOWN ☐ OTHER
NARRATIVE	

TIME	P	R	B/P	TREATMENT	RESPONSE/COMMENTS

- To save your log, click on the disk icon. To print your log, click on the printer icon.
- Click **Menu** to return to the summary menu.
- Click **Exit** to close the program, or **Restart** to continue with another lesson.

EXERCISE 2

Summary Activity

Time: 10 minutes

11. How do you believe you handled this call?

12. Do you think you would change your actions if given the opportunity to complete the call again?

    If you said *yes*, what would you change and how do you think those changes would affect the patient?

- Review your log with your instructor to see how it compares with the recommended care found in the implementation manual.

13. How did your care compare with what was recommended?

14. After reviewing the call, would you change anything on a subsequent call of this nature? Explain your answer.

Ambulance Operations

👓 **Reading Assignment:** Read Chapter 26, Ambulance Operations, in *EMT Prehospital Care,* Fourth Edition.

Case 5: 40-year-old male—vomiting blood

Objectives:

On completion of this lesson, the student will be able to perform the following:

- Relate the need for specialty resources for this case.
- Describe appropriate helicopter safety procedures as they relate to this case.
- Discuss principles of safe ambulance operation.

EXERCISE 1

 CD-ROM Activity

 Time: 10 minutes

→ • Sign into the software by entering your name in the name tag and clicking **Enter**.
   • Choose the case by clicking on *Case 5: 40-year-old male—vomiting blood*.
   • Listen to the dispatch, or read it in the right panel (or both).
   • Click **Start**, and watch the entire video. Once the video has concluded, you are "on scene."
   • Read the history log on the right side of the screen.

1. Does this call meet the general requirements for air medical transport?

2. Are there specific requirements for air medical transport within your local region that you would take into consideration on this call?

3. Can you identify a suitable landing zone, based on what you saw in the video?

4. What additional resources may be needed to set up the landing zone?

5. When the helicopter lands, describe how and when you will approach the aircraft.

6. If the air ambulance is not available, should you transport the patient with or without lights and sirens? Explain your answer.

7. Describe how you will proceed through intersections.

8. What are the laws within your state with regard to ambulance operations in emergency mode?

→   • Click **Quit Case**, and you will be taken to the summary menu.
   • Click **Exit** to close the program, or **Restart** to continue with another lesson.

LESSON 27

Geriatric Emergencies

✐ **Reading Assignment:** Read Chapter 31, Geriatric Emergencies, in *EMT Prehospital Care,* Fourth Edition.

Other Relevant Chapters:
- Chapter 2, Well-Being of the EMT
- Chapter 7, Patient Assessment
- Chapter 9, Documentation
- Chapter 10, General Pharmacology
- Chapter 11, Respiratory Emergencies
- Chapter 12, Cardiovascular Emergencies

Case 14: 65-year-old male—difficulty breathing

Objectives:
On completion of this lesson, the student will be able to perform the following:
- Describe modifications in assessment and treatment for the geriatric patient.
- Perform appropriate interventions for the patient with dyspnea.
- Describe characteristics and method of administration of nitroglycerin.
- Document this case appropriately.

EXERCISE 1

 CD-ROM Activity

 Time: 15 minutes

- Sign into the software by entering your name in the name tag and clicking **Enter**.
- Choose the case by clicking on *Case 14: 65-year-old male—difficulty breathing*.
- Listen to the dispatch, or read it in the right panel (or both).
- Click **Start**, and watch the entire video. Once the video has concluded, you are "on scene."
- Read the history log on the right side of the screen.
- Perform your assessments and interventions using the buttons in the left panel. When you have determined that it is appropriate to begin transporting your patient to the hospital, click the **Load Patient** button. Continue your assessments and interventions en route to the hospital. When you have finished treating your patient, click the **Unload Patient** button. You will be taken to the summary menu.
- Click the **Log** button on the summary menu, and review your patient care as you answer the following questions.

  1. Did you notice the dog barking in the background? How could that influence your call? What actions might you need to take to address this situation?

  2. What was the significance of this patient's home oxygen?

  3. List at least four possible causes of his difficulty breathing.

4. What is the most likely cause of this patient's dyspnea? Describe the factors that led you to this determination.

5. Complete the following information related to the administration of nitroglycerin to this patient.

   a. What are the trade names for nitroglycerin?

   b. How does nitroglycerin work to relieve chest pain?

   c. If the patient's blood pressure (BP) drops below 100 mm Hg after you give nitroglycerin, what should you do?

   d. List three things you should check on the patient's prescribed nitroglycerin container before you give it.

   e. How many doses of nitroglycerin can be given?

   f. From whom must you get permission to administer nitroglycerin?

   g. Nitroglycerin is administered to patients who have what signs or symptoms?

h. List at least four reasons you would NOT give nitroglycerin.

i. What is the correct dose of nitroglycerin?

j. By what route is nitroglycerin given?

k. What should be assessed after nitroglycerin has been given?

6. List nonpharmacologic interventions for this patient, and explain why you used them.

7. For each of the physical findings below, describe how you would assess the finding and its significance.

Finding	Assessment Technique	Significance
Crackles (rales) in the lungs		
Pedal edema		

8. List at least two age-related changes that you notice in this patient as you watch the initial video clip.

9. Describe how age-related changes may affect patient care or assessment in each of the following examples.

Action to Be Performed	Body System	Effect on Assessment or Patient Care
Blood pressure assessment	Cardiovascular	
Standing patient to move to stretcher	Cardiovascular	
Respiratory rate assessment	Respiratory	

10. Complete a patient care report (PCR) for this call. (Use the following blank or one your instructor has given you.)

CHIEF COMPLAINT	
CURRENT MEDICATIONS	☐ NONE KNOWN
ALLERGIES (MEDICATIONS)	☐ NONE KNOWN
MEDICAL HISTORY	☐ MI ☐ CHF ☐ COPD ☐ ↑ BP ☐ DIABETES ☐ CANCER ☐ NONE KNOWN ☐ OTHER
NARRATIVE	

TIME	P	R	B/P	TREATMENT	RESPONSE/COMMENTS

• To save your log, click on the disk icon. To print your log, click on the printer icon.

• Click **Menu** to return to the summary menu.

• Click **Exit** to close the program, or **Restart** to continue with another lesson.

EXERCISE 2

 Summary Activity

 **Time:** 10 minutes

11. How do you believe you handled this call?

12. Do you think you would change your actions if given the opportunity to complete the call again?

   If you said *yes*, what would you change and how do you think those changes would affect the patient?

 • Review your log with your instructor to see how it compares with the recommended care found in the implementation manual.

13. How did your care compare with what was recommended?

14. After reviewing the call, would you change anything on a subsequent call of this nature? Explain your answer.